THE PRACTICE OF EYE MOVEMENT DESENSITIZATION

To Sarah
22 Feb 2023
Alan
Hassard

THE PRACTICE OF EYE MOVEMENT DESENSITIZATION

Alan Hassard

Matador
Unit E2 Airfield Business Park,
Harrison Road, Market Harborough,
Leicestershire. LE16 7UL
Tel: 0116 2792299
Email: books@troubador.co.uk
Web: www.troubador.co.uk/matador
Twitter: @matadorbooks

ISBN 978 1800465 527

British Library Cataloguing in Publication Data.
A catalogue record for this book is available from the British Library.

Printed and bound in the UK by TJ Books LTD, Padstow, Cornwall
Typeset in 10pt Minion Pro by Troubador Publishing Ltd, Leicester, UK

Matador is an imprint of Troubador Publishing Ltd

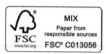

For my parents

Albert James Hassard (1922–2005)

Patricia Mary (Faldo) Hassard (1928–2020)
The strongest person I ever knew

CONTENTS

7 DIFFERENT TREATMENT TARGETS 111

1. A BRIEF INTRODUCTION

1.1 WHY DO THIS THING?

Thank you for starting this book. I will explain why I wrote it and why I would like you to continue with it, given how many books on eye movement desensitization there are these days. A book like this must be as objective as possible, but some minimal personal statement is required. When I start a book I read the author's biography and introduction to get the author's experience and point of view. I give the backstory here to explain my bias on procedure and why we should use eye movement desensitization.

I remember attending a lecture on plastic surgery for burns and other military injuries at Derriford Hospital, Plymouth. This must have been late 1990, as we prepared to receive casualties from the first Gulf War. The lecture was on skin grafting, in which the innate repair functions of the body's surface are exploited by taking skin from one site on the patient's body to the face or other visible injury. I left the lecture wondering what my own trade, clinical psychology, could offer that was that good. I remembered an odd report claiming that distress images could be affected by systematic eye movements. I had dismissed this as too weird to be true.

In 1987, I had been pleasantly surprised when I was appointed to a job in Plymouth. I was the only candidate, which is a good, but not foolproof, method of seeking employment. I had narrowly survived my passage through a clinical psychology school at a northern university, for reasons I have now forgotten. Except this reason: at this school, I had been baffled and wrongfooted by the apparent inability of my teachers to spell out procedure.

Previously, in the early 1970s, I was a biochemistry technician in an immunology research laboratory in south London, run by a drug company that now exists only as a medical research foundation. Lab techs are taught that procedure is everything. I could rarely find a procedure specified in clinical psychology. One exception was psychometric testing, where the procedure was specified in a manual. No doubt these tests are now on tablet computers. Otherwise, at that time, only the behaviour therapists and cognitive therapists explained what to do and justified their effectiveness by running trials, not with rhetoric or good intentions. I could never understand the psychodynamic idea that exposure to sympathetic conversation and some mysterious quality in my personality could cure or help the patient. A colleague once attributed my success to some virtue of my powerful personality, rather than eye movements. I fear she did not know my personality as well as I did. I never understood the idea that my own personality had any such virtue. One patient described to me previous therapy sessions in which she sat opposite the therapist for an hour, but not much was said. Many cigarettes were consumed. No doubt this was some kind of existential therapy.

I hope I am not mischaracterizing this. Of course, people do move on when they are assisted by an attentive listener to articulate and hear the self-talk in their mind. At the simplest level the listener can be anybody with the time, but for anything more, a good psychotherapist is needed to interlocute and catalyse this. I have even done this myself, I hope with good effect. However, I thought that the hard-earned privilege of a National Health Service psychology job meant you had to explain what you did. I still think this, and this conviction seems to have resulted in this whole book.

The job involved a new virus epidemic, discovered in San Francisco, and then appearing in Plymouth. Because human immunodeficiency virus (HIV) is mostly sexually transmitted, the genito-urinary medicine department was dealing with this issue. This infection might present with memory or behavioural problems, so a psychologist job was funded. The epidemic was immunological and I was probably the only psychologist in Britain with experience in immunology. I probably still am. It turned out that psychiatric presentations were rare, and prevented by improving medication.

After the lecture on plastic surgery, I reread Francine Shapiro's protocol report, and noted that it referenced a randomized controlled trial. I retrieved this and was impressed.

I know there are problems with this and later trials, but I was impressed. Now, I find it extraordinary that Dr Shapiro managed to publish these reports. There was then no training available in Britain, so I wrote a protocol, as I had been taught in the lab. The first official training in Britain was in 1994. My attempts to do cognitive therapy with a work accident victim had not been helpful. I asked her if she could see images of the accident. She became distressed. Lesson of 1991: ask for the bad pictures first. She agreed to try this new method. Most readers of this book know the next stage. You have to keep a straight face when the distressing images and bad thoughts reduce that fast. It occurred to me that I might be in the right place at the right time to start this new procedure. The genito-urinary medicine clinic took the sexual assault and misadventure victims. Perhaps they had distress images in their heads that could be made to disappear like this. I discussed this with the Health Advisor team, and showed them some examples...

That original protocol has been rewritten and expanded over the years since then. It spent many years lying fallow, while I collected facts and wrote lists. I dealt with my own life events and told myself nobody read books. Then I would recollect that I read books, so maybe other people did also. One day I realized the Life Rule 'finish what you start' applied and pulled it together. You are about to read the result.

Why do eye movement desensitization anyway? What is the point in replacing ten sessions of whatever therapy with ten sessions of eye movement desensitization? Why should that impress the clinic budget holder? It must have some benefit to justify it. The position taken in this book is that we replace ten sessions of whatever therapy with five sessions of eye movement desensitization. We can do this only if we deprecate the advice in many manuals on our subject to do other things. If we consider the canonical account, by which I mean the third edition of Dr Shapiro's book, we find many recommendations. When do we do these things? It appears the clients in California tolerate several appointments doing other distress control procedures before any eye movement therapy happens. They keep logs of their emotions and will take advice about their lifestyle.

My patients will not give me that much time. They do not keep logs; they have childcare issues or serious medical illnesses or chronic pain. They consent to treatment, then do not attend or drop out after one, two or three good sessions, no doubt assuming the treatment is finished. They do not always tell me the truth, an issue noted in the final chapter. In my hospital clinics, there is the continual pressure of new patients. The minimalist and utilitarian version of eye movement desensitization procedure given here has developed in that context.

May I be explicit on one point in this book, in case the reader might miss it. This is the importance of eye movement desensitization in medical patients. This book is a report on some 30 years of experience of our method on patients in a medical hospital, not a psychiatry team or psychological therapy clinic. This is mostly in the sexual health clinic, but also the pain clinic and for intensive care survivors. After these three clinics, I suspect most candidates are in the diabetes, cancer, cardiology and gastroenterology clinics. I suspect at least a quarter of medical patients, and perhaps up to half, could benefit from eye movement desensitization. However, most of the bad life events reported by such candidates may not concern those medical misfortunes, but will be other distressing memories and triggers that are clogging up their working memory. This prevents them from coping with their illness or chronic pain, stopping unwise sexual behaviour, fulfilling their whole potential or spending less in the supermarket.

And here's another issue. Many colleagues still do not show any interest in eye movement desensitization after 30 years. Why is this, given that it reduces therapy time?

I have struggled to understand this since 1991. One explanation is the problem of unbalanced randomized controlled trials noted in the final chapter. There is something more. It is something about people's implicit models or theories of mind or behaviour. Such assumptions are more powerful than I anticipated, or at least people do not allow for them. In this time, I have attempted to read a few books on theoretical psychology or philosophy of mind, but have achieved only a limited understanding of the issue. One thing has stuck and that is the importance of sorting things into the right categories. For a simple example, oranges and apples are in the fruit category. Bread and cakes are baking. We know these two categories are separate. Apples and cakes are not in the same category unless we combine them in a recipe category, such as

Devon apple cake. The point is that we are thinking about membership of categories or sets.

The categories that appear later in this book are more abstract and the sets of objects or events more difficult to define. I will later say it is helpful to divide psychological treatment methods into procedural or rhetorical. Claiming that eye movement desensitization is in the procedural category enables us to predict that difficulties in treatment are best resolved with changes in procedure.

We should know if a distress memory is episodic or semantic. An episodic memory is the memory of one episode or event. A semantic memory is a general memory caused by repetition of the event. Eye movement desensitization works on semantic memory and does not require us to work through every episode in a difficult life history. If a patient is assaulted or persecuted in some way every weekend for 10 years, there are not 520 separate episodes. If there were, it might take us 1,000 treatment sessions, instead of three or four.

Asking for the story without distinguishing between episodic and semantic memory may lead to a judgement of complexity. I have often seen the opinion that a case is too complex for eye movement desensitization. This may stem from concern that the patient will produce some narrative surprises during treatment. This risk can be eliminated, or at least reduced, by a robust request to list all bad life events and by enquiring whether everything has been asked and answered, at the end of the first session. If we stay in the procedural category, we recall that in other fields, such as physics and biology, it has been discovered that complexity can result from the repetition of simple rules. Perhaps we can undo complexity by the repetition of procedural rules.

Eye movement desensitization is not a narrative therapy. Narrative therapy is a subset of rhetorical therapies. Eye movement desensitization does not require knowing or exploring the patient's complete life history, although writing a bad life events list is advised. Most of this book addresses procedure. I do not claim that narrative is to be dismissed. You have read some of mine above. Also, a note of caution: this is about adults. Using eye movement desensitization with children requires developing the story. Perhaps children have more episodic memory than semantic because they have been here for a shorter time.

I will introduce the idea of determinism. For our purposes here, this means an implicit belief that behaviour is caused, or mostly caused, by one particular antecedent cause. We can change the behaviour if we change this cause. This might be, for example, emotions, cognition, language or images. An implicit belief in linguistic or emotional determinism, for example, may mean that an image-based procedure is regarded as inferior or even impossible. I suspect that this implicit bias to cognitive, or at least linguistic, determinism is because we all self-talk. We all introspect, so that must be the explanation. Once we understand that the words in our head are not those of gods, demons, river spirits or ancestors, but self-instructions from our experience of the world seen from the point of view of our brain, then we assume that both our, and other people's, behaviour can be modified by self-talk. And of course it can.

The linguistic determination of behaviour means we can write and read this book, or instruct people to keep two metres apart in a respiratory virus pandemic.

However, there is another way. Imagine there is a three-dimensional network of 80 billion neurons in your brain. This is difficult to imagine, but it is the reality. This thing is really there between your ears. Memory information is held in this network and we use the metaphor of activation or energy to understand how. Simplify the image by transforming it into a two-dimensional network. You can transform images in your mind. Now energy information can be represented by bumps or peaks in the network.

The place the bump is sitting is called the node. Like any physical system, the node has a limit on the amount of energy information it can hold. If the node becomes overloaded, we experience the overflowing node as a repeated flashback or memory image. If too much energy information sits in one node, then the network is strained. A strained node causes it's owner to become distressed. We can measure the strain with a simple zero-to-ten ordinal scale. Perhaps we can reduce the strain by gently tapping on the network or nudging it in some way. If we can find a way of doing this, then the network may go back to that minimum energy state where it really wants to be. Perhaps this tendency to equilibrium is something like the innate repair mechanism I was looking for when I left the plastic surgery lecture.

This discomfort with image-based methods of psychological therapy goes back to systematic desensitization in the 1960s. I once demonstrated eye movement desensitization to a colleague. I have to say it did not go well, and it later transpired that the patient had stalled on a flashforward that triggered a panic. My colleague was not impressed and her objection was: 'why did you not talk to her?' Answer: because eye movement desensitization is a procedural method based on image determinism. It is not in the category rhetorical methods, based on cognitive determinism. At least, here it is not.

I have tried to write as simply as possible, but not simpler. The author is asking the reader to commit to the task of reading the book. It seems both polite and wise to make that task as easy as can be contrived. Why should I overload the reader's working memory? Most psychology writing in journals and books is terrible stuff. Why is it so turgid, with redundant clauses and contextual information? Why do they say 'paradigm' when they mean method? Why do they say 'methodology' when they mean method? Surely psychologists are not fooled by language as a status symbol or a rhetorical device to define the in-group? I once discussed this with a colleague from Germany. How did she cope with psychology English as a second language? She said it was not so bad and much of the vocabulary was the same. I think she was just being polite. I have also eliminated most acronyms, except in the sleep-stage diagrams, the index and identifying some common usage in the text. I think they are just another obfuscation and turn the text into some sinister n-back working memory game.

Let us review the chapters, to light the way ahead. Chapter 2 considers diagnostic definitions and attempts to explain and unpack the idea of post-traumatic stress disorder. Perhaps some of the confusion about eye movement desensitization starts as confusion about post-traumatic stress disorder. Chapter 3 classifies memory and memory failures. The brain is not a memory device. It does not store a reliable narrative. It is a navigation device, containing a map or model of the world of it's owner. It collects information to map, navigate and predict the owner's world. Chapter 4 describes the images, cognitions and emotion names used to label the bad core affect feelings that it is our mission to eliminate. We visit some helpful ideas about emotion and the predictive function of memory.

Chapter 5 concerns measurement. This is a dry subject, but required for eye movement desensitization as advocated here. A decrease in distress score shows boundaries between images. If the image memory is semantic, then this boundary may not be otherwise apparent, as in the case of an episode.

Chapter 6 is the original protocol. As it expanded, I listed different targets and problems separately, making Chapters 7 and 8. Method (x), variations of image or target (y) and troubleshooting problems (z) are described separately. Imagine that each is represented by the x, y and z co-ordinates of a three-dimensional space. A treatment session could go anywhere in that space.

Chapters 9 and 10 attempt to explain eye movement desensitization, first considering working memory and then comparison with rapid eye movement sleep. The working memory explanation works best. I have not reviewed or compared other explanations of our problem. The reader can find them in other journals and books. I want to use my space to work out my own ideas. Chapter 11 is an informal series of notes, or leftover matters, not all logically connected. These are things that are of interest to me and, I hope, the reader.

1.2 ACKNOWLEDGEMENTS AND DISCLAIMER

These introductions must contain the author's thanks. Many authors find a lot of people to thank. In one book, I found a list of people to whom the author owed gratitude that was four pages long. How did the author keep track of all these teachers and mentors? Perhaps there was a database. In my case, my professional network has always been modest and volatile. However, I have discovered that not everybody has read *Effectiveness and Efficiency*, and not everybody supports innovation and improvement; or, to use the current polite term, wants to improve the patient experience. I owe a vote of thanks to those who do. I must thank the health advisers, doctors, nurses and other colleagues of the Genito-Urinary Medicine Department of Derriford Hospital, Plymouth (now re-branded as SHiP, meaning Sexual Health in Plymouth), for their support for eye movement desensitization since 1991. I must also thank the patients, whose identity is a legal secret. Outside genito-urinary medicine, I should thank David Mulhall, Ron Wood, Dinah Jenkins and Wendy van der Niet for patient and supportive discussions.

I should also thank those eye movement desensitization colleagues I have met, listened to and discussed with at meetings and peer supervision groups since 1991. I did not record or remember all their names, but perhaps that is where the four pages of names come from. I apologize if any of their ideas appear unreferenced or uncredited here. I do not remember every discussion and I am taking a relaxed attitude to references.

The Disclaimer Clauses

This book is for educational and dialectical purposes only. Also: 'trigger warning', for those readers not yet aware that this book concerns desensitizing such triggers. This book contains explicit trauma stories, some of which are explicitly sexual. Readers who want to learn how to desensitize such triggers for their patients should continue. All case stories here are abstracted, have details changed or are combinations of similar cases.

For the Patient

If you are considering this treatment, you are welcome to read this book. But this is not a self-help book. This book is not intended to be a substitute for professional clinical advice. You should not use this information to diagnose or treat a health problem without consulting a healthcare provider who is qualified in your jurisdiction. Please consult your healthcare provider with any questions or concerns you may have regarding your condition.

For the Therapist

Eye movement desensitization is a physiologically accelerated form of cognitive behavioural therapy. Or, at least, it should be. Therefore, previous experience and understanding of cognitive behavioural methods is an asset. Eye movement desensitization requires a specific assessment and measurement of the flashback or target, similar to a good cognitive behavioural method. In the British context, which the author knows, eye movement desensitization is used by clinical and counselling psychologists, psychiatric nurse-therapists and psychiatrists. Other people with qualifications, at least to degree level, in psychotherapy or counselling may qualify. No doubt this will be similar in other clinical jurisdictions.

Practitioners without such professional qualifications, training or experience should not start eye movement desensitization after reading this account. Eye movement desensitization should not be performed by amateurs, volunteers, 'holistic practitioners', hypnotherapist or para-professionals. My resolution to write about eye movement desensitization as simply as possible does not make it a simple matter. I advise against doing it over a video link, at least as advocated in this book. However, in the abnormal circumstances of the coronavirus pandemic lockdown, we have attempted this with some success.

1.3 BRIEFING THE PATIENT

This is the patient information leaflet I use. You can copy or adapt this section. I include it here to introduce the method advocated in this book and some of the issues it raises.

Eye Movement Desensitization and Reprocessing

Information for patients

Please read this carefully. EMDR helps people with trauma memories, disturbing experiences, stress and anxiety. The EMDR therapist will need to know four things about your problem:

1. The flashback or image
2. The distressing thoughts that come with the flashback
3. The physical feelings that go with the flashback
4. How distressed you feel during the flashback. The therapist will ask you to measure how distressed you feel using an imaginary ruler from zero to ten. Zero means that you feel OK about it. Ten means you are as distressed as you can be.

Talking about bad memories can be distressing. The therapist needs to know only the first flashback to start the treatment. EMDR is best done in a business-like and clinical fashion, to get you through the procedure. You may not remember part of the trauma and the therapist will discuss this with you.

The therapist will ask you to think about the flashback. At the same time, you will track his/her hand (or a stick) so your eyes move from side to side. The therapist will do this in sets of about 25 movements. If you find this distressing and difficult at first, it should get easier. Other methods are available if you have a problem moving your eyes.

At the end of each set, please blank out the flashback and take a deep breath. Then report any changes in the flashback and the distress number. As you go through sets, the flashback seems to get further away from you and the distress decreases. Usually, people say the flashback is becoming misty or foggy. The image seems further away from them, like something they saw in a film. Next it will feel like the flashback is difficult to concentrate on. At the end, they can remember what happened but without distress. On average, this takes about 15 sets per flashback.

At some point, the next flashback will come to your attention. Tell the therapist even if it is difficult or embarrassing. All flashbacks you report should be treated with EMDR. The average number of flashbacks is seven. Most people need three or four treatment sessions.

Sometimes people do not want to lose the flashback completely. For example, they may want to remember somebody who died in an accident. If you want to keep part of an image, but at a level that is less distressing, let the therapist know when you want to stop.

EMDR induces permanent results, as far as we know. There are two exceptions to this. Flashbacks may return if the patient is reminded with enough force of the bad thing that happened. An example of this is if a woman meets the man who assaulted her. The second exception is if the patient does not tell the therapist about all the flashbacks or bad things that have happened.

There are three possible problems during treatment:
1. It can be slow to start in the first two or three sets. You may feel a bit strange at first, until you understand what is happening.
2. Sometimes the flashback and the distressing thought will not make sense together. If this happens, the therapist will

ask 'What are you telling yourself now?' and then carry on with this new thought.

3. Sometimes people remember something else distressing. They may feel the pain or sensations from a painful medical treatment or a physical or sexual assault. This is upsetting, but usually lasts only a few minutes at worst. This means that EMDR has reached the most important part of the memory. You must then continue EMDR for the new flashback. You should agree before the treatment starts that if this happens, you will continue EMDR.

After the session, please remember five things:

1. You may feel light-headed and tired afterwards. You may not feel like going back to work. A few patients have reported headaches. If this happens, do whatever you usually do to deal with a headache.

2. Treating bad memories does not mean that your problem was trivial or imagined.

3. When the treatment works you can expect improvements. Until the EMDR is finished, any improvement after one session may reverse. You may remember other bad memories. If this happens, report them back to the therapist, who will give you further treatment.

4. If you have panic attacks, you may have a panic between sessions. You may become anxious that you will have another panic attack. Tell the therapist this is happening. Solving this problem may require several appointments close together.

5. Do not drive a car for 30 minutes after each treatment session. You may need to allow for this in your travel arrangements.

Attending Appointments

About half the people who start EMDR do not finish. Some drop out before treatment starts. Others drop out after some successful sessions, perhaps thinking they have finished. Treatment is not finished until the therapist has checked that all flashbacks have been treated successfully. Unfinished treatment may result in continuing problems.

If you change your mind about EMDR, do not miss your appointment. If you attend, you can discuss any doubts or other issues. Patients who miss appointments without notice not only forgo the appointment, but they prevent us from giving it to somebody else who needs it. This means two people lose a treatment session. If you do not wish to attend an appointment, please cancel it as soon as you can.

2. POST-TRAUMATIC STRAIN DISORDER

2.1 DEFINITION

Here I consider definitions of post-traumatic stress disorder, argue that caution is needed with this diagnosis and advocate that we should rename it post-traumatic *strain* disorder. When bad things happen to people, some (but not all) of these victims develop psychological disorder or illness of various kinds. This is generally called post-traumatic stress disorder, but may be another form of anxiety, depression or panic.

Classification of mental illness or emotional disorder is required because we are obliged to help more than one person during our career. Assume we develop a theory concerning the problems or illness of the first patient, who we will call Alice. This theory, which we might call a formulation or narrative, is helpful to Alice. How does this help our second patient (Bob)? We could devise a second theory, but it might be better to ask what Alice and Bob have in common. If both have symptoms in common then we could use this to identify a category of patients. This could be a diagnostic category that indicates the best treatment. This means that we can help or cure some or all of these patients. It also enables us to discuss Alice's problems with Alice, or with our colleagues.

There are two definitions of post-traumatic stress disorder, considering adults only. The first is from the *Diagnostic and Statistical Manual of Mental Disorders of the American Psychiatric Association* (DSM-5) [1]. Below is my summary of the first five symptom groups. Not all items from the list are required. The patient needs either one or two from each group to qualify. Also, these symptoms must be present six months after the event, but may take longer to appear. The symptoms last longer than one month. They cause distress or impairment. Symptoms are not caused by medication, substance use or other illness.

Criterion A

The person experienced or was threatened with death, serious injury or sexual violence. This may be one or more events. Indirect exposure through media is excluded.

1. By direct exposure.
2. By witnessing, in person.

3. Indirectly, by information that somebody close to the person was exposed to such an event.
4. By professional exposure to such events or information.

Criterion B

One symptom of re-experiencing the event.

1. Recurrent or intrusive memories.
2. Nightmares.
3. Dissociative reactions (e.g. flashbacks), which may be brief episodes of loss of consciousness.
4. Distress after exposure to reminders.
5. Physiological reactivity after exposure to related stimuli.

Criterion C

One symptom of avoiding distressing reminders.

1. Related thoughts or feelings.
2. External reminders, such as places.

Criterion D

Two symptoms of negative cognitions and mood that began or worsened after the event.

1. Inability to recall key features of the traumatic event, usually dissociative amnesia (excluding head injury, alcohol or drugs).

2. Persistent and distorted negative thoughts about oneself or the world.
3. Blame self or others for the event or consequences.
4. Negative emotions, such as fear, horror, anger, guilt or shame.
5. Decreased interest in previous activities.
6. Feeling isolated from others.
7. Reduced positive emotions.

Criterion E

Two symptoms of alterations in arousal and reactivity.

1. Appearance of increase in arousal and reactivity.
2. Irritable or aggressive behaviour.
3. Self-destructive or reckless behaviour.
4. Hyper-vigilance.
5. Exaggerated startle response.
6. Loss of concentration.
7. Sleep disturbance.

The patient may also report dissociative symptoms. Dissociative symptoms, or dissociation, is discussed elsewhere, but here covers two possible symptoms:

1. **Depersonalization:** reporting being an observer of, or detached from, oneself and other people.
2. **Derealization:** a report of unreality, distance, or distortion.

Note the 'statistical' nature of this definition. If a patient meets all the criteria except physiological arousal, does this mean there is no post-traumatic stress disorder? That might seem unfair.

These criteria make statistical and epidemiological sense, but are not useful clinically. If eye movement desensitization is recommended for post-traumatic stress disorder, does this mean only those patients that check the list exactly? Obviously, it does not.

The second definition is from the International Statistical Classification of Diseases and Related Health Problems, Revision 10, of the World Health Organisation (ICD-10) [2]. A series of disorders is classified under the title of 'Reaction to severe stress and adjustment disorders'. Below is my précis of this definition. This describes the syndrome and introduces vulnerability factors and other symptoms.

(ICD-10) Post-traumatic stress disorder is a response to a stressful event or situation (of either brief or long duration) of an exceptionally threatening or catastrophic nature, which is likely to cause pervasive distress in almost anyone. Predisposing factors, such as personality traits or previous history of neurotic illness, may lower the threshold for the development of the syndrome but do not explain its occurrence. Typical features include episodes of repeated reliving of the trauma in intrusive memories ('flashbacks'), dreams or nightmares, a sense of 'numbness' and emotional blunting, detachment from other people, unresponsiveness to surroundings, and avoidance of activities and situations reminiscent of the trauma. There is usually a state of autonomic hyperarousal with hypervigilance, enhanced startle reaction, and insomnia. Anxiety and depression commonly occur. Suicidal ideation may occur. The course is fluctuating but recovery occurs in most cases. In a small proportion of cases the condition becomes chronic over many years, causing an enduring personality change.

Also included here is 'acute stress reaction' and 'adjustment disorders'. Acute stress reaction has symptoms such as anxiety or anger, which appear soon after the event and last a few days. Adjustment disorders are reactions such as anxiety or depression in response to distressing life events. They last about six months. Another trauma response is described as 'enduring personality change after a catastrophic experience'. This is a response to severe trauma events, without any other cause such as brain disease. The patient suffers a chronic personality change, which should be validated by an informant. Symptoms are impairment of social functioning, estrangement and a chronic feeling of being threatened.

2.2 PANICS

Other psychological disorders, such as other anxiety or depression, can be caused by the experience of bad life events. As an example, panic is defined here. A panic is a surge of intense anxiety or discomfort that peaks in minutes from previous state of calm or lower anxiety. Four symptoms from a list of thirteen are needed to qualify:

1. Palpitations or faster heart rate
2. Sweating
3. Trembling or shaking
4. Shortness of breath
5. A choking feeling
6. Chest pain or discomfort
7. Nausea or abdominal distress
8. Feeling dizzy, light-headed or faint
9. Chills or heat sensations
10. Paresthesia (numbness or tingling sensations)
11. Derealization (feelings of unreality) or depersonalization (being detached from oneself)
12. Fear of losing control or going crazy
13. Fear of dying

The patient may report other symptoms, such as crying, head or neck pain, or thoughts about an imminent catastrophe such as loss of control or death. These symptoms are not required for the panic definition. Panic can be part of a psychological problem. For example, a report of agoraphobia may be better defined as staying in to avoid an anticipated panic attack outside. The patient may report severe anxiety attacks that do not score four of the above. Panic symptoms without bad thoughts may be reported. Panics may have an originating event, or some event given that status by the patient. Such post-traumatic panic is then similar to post-traumatic stress disorder. However, the originating event can be the first panic attack, not any other life event. Assessment for eye movement desensitization enquires after the first, worst, most recent and future panics. The first is often also the worst.

Panic attacks can be a problem in treatment. Some patients may panic when focusing on a flashback.

2.3 WHAT CAUSES POST-TRAUMATIC STRESS DISORDER?

We could answer that trauma causes post-traumatic stress disorder, but this makes problems that need to be unpacked. Perhaps this argument is both circular and narrative. Psychological illness following a trauma event is called this, but perhaps requires other causes. Perhaps similar anxiety and depression, with distressing images, can occur after an originating event that sounds less traumatic to the listener. Perhaps no originating event is reported. How do we discover the cause of an illness? This complex subject is simplified here by considering two indicators of causation [3]. These are dose response and specificity. Dose response means that the probability of the illness increases with the amount of the pathogenic agent the patient experiences. Examples of this can be found for post-traumatic stress disorder and some are given below.

Is post-traumatic stress disorder specifically caused by trauma events? Our patients will tell us their problem started with a bad life event. Are they right? They are, in the personal narrative sense, but to develop a good theory that might help other patients, we need to consider other possibilities. There are four possible combinations of events, shown logically in the Latin square below.

Bad life events happen and cause psychological illness.	Bad life events happen but do not cause psychological illness.
Bad life events do not happen but there is psychological illness.	Bad life events do not happen and there is no psychological illness.

2.4 NOT EVERYBODY GETS POST-TRAUMATIC STRESS DISORDER

If all victims of trauma events get post-traumatic stress disorder, then maybe trauma events are a specific cause of the disorder. If we can show that not all victims proceed to the disorder, then maybe other causes are needed as well. Following up victims of bad life events and measuring the effects is a major research industry. The general result is that not everybody gets post-traumatic stress disorder. Some people get other issues and some people get better. Other events in the subject's history may encourage psychological illness and these are referred to as risk factors. These are properties of the life event or the victim that increase the probability that post-traumatic stress disorder or other psychological problems will develop. A medical analogy is that tuberculosis is defined by infection by *Mycobacterium tuberculosis*. However, we can find people who are infected but not ill. It requires additional factors, such as bad social conditions, bad nutrition or human immunodeficiency virus infection, to encourage the bacteria. Some examples follow.

A survey of traumatic life events and post-traumatic stress disorder was made by a household survey of the population of south-east London [4]. Face-to-face interviews took place in randomly chosen households, with translators for those who could not speak English. There were 1,698 respondents in total. Most of these people (78%) had experienced at least one bad life event. However, the prevalence of post-traumatic stress disorder was 5.5%. Males reported more physical violence and females reported more sexual assault. There was a dose effect. Respondents with one event had a prevalence of 1.9%, rising progressively to 21.6% for those with five and 27.2% for those with six. Prevalence was larger when income, educational status or employment status was lower.

Another epidemiological study showed a dose response [5]. A population of 7,400 subjects were questioned for issues such as psychiatric disorders and drug use. Subjects answered these questions on a laptop computer under confidential conditions:

1. Has anyone talked to you in a sexual way that made you feel uncomfortable?
2. Has anyone touched you, or got you to touch them, in a sexual way without your consent?
3. Has anyone had sexual intercourse with you without your consent?

The bad effects for all assessed disorders increased up this scale of sexual impropriety. Here are two examples. For post-traumatic stress disorder, this increased three, four and eight times, for each question, from the background population level. For depression, the values were two, three and five times more. Similarly, these subjects were divided into those who experienced the event either below the age of 16, above the age of 16, or both sides of age 16. Those who experienced the event both sides of age 16 had higher psychopathology. Note that we have dose response but lose specificity. There was increased risk for depression, anxiety, generalized anxiety, panic, phobia, obsessive compulsive disorder, drug and alcohol dependence, post-traumatic stress disorder and eating disorders.

Some factors increase the risk of post-traumatic stress. Pain is one example. Various epidemiological reports can be found showing that chronic pain and post-traumatic stress disorder overlap in the population. This is not considered further here, but pain is considered later as a treatment issue. A small hippocampus is such a risk factor.

2.5 THE HIPPOCAMPUS

The hippocampus is a brain structure sitting approximately between the ears. 'Hippocampus' is Latin for 'seahorse', named to remind the brain anatomist of the shape. It is a symmetrical structure with a right and a left side. Imagine two seahorses with their tails intertwined in the centre of your brain, with the heads pointing forward. They bend round so that each head lies closer to each of the ears. A meta-analysis – that is, a statistical summary of a number of reports and subjects – showed that the volume of the hippocampus tends to be smaller in patients with post-traumatic stress disorder, compared with non-patients. Also, more severe post-traumatic stress disorder was associated with small hippocampus volume [6].

The problem then becomes this question: does post-traumatic stress disorder cause a small hippocampus or does a small hippocampus cause post-traumatic stress disorder? There is a clever investigation of this [7]. Identical male twin pairs were recruited; one of whom had served in the Vietnam War and the other had not. There were 17 twin pairs where the military twin had post-traumatic stress disorder and 23 pairs where the military twin did not have post-traumatic stress disorder. It is likely that identical twins have a similar-sized hippocampus. The brains of these subjects were scanned and hippocampal volume correlated at 0.9 in the twin pairs. A correlation value of 1.0 would mean the hippocampi were the same size in each twin. In the post-traumatic stress disorder cases, severity correlated inversely (at –0.54) with hippocampal volume. Smaller hippocampus, more post-traumatic stress disorder.

Also, symptom severity in the military twin correlated with hippocampal volume in the civilian twin. Since the civilian twin did not experience combat, or otherwise have post-traumatic stress disorder, then the small hippocampus existed in the military twin before the post-traumatic stress disorder developed. Therefore a small hippocampus is a physiological risk factor for post-traumatic stress disorder. A 5ml hippocampus is less helpful in overcoming trauma than a 10ml hippocampus. Clearly this is a genetic factor, but further discussion of genetics is omitted here.

2.6 PSYCHOLOGICAL ILLNESS BUT NO BAD LIFE EVENTS

Post-traumatic stress disorder is the only mental or emotional illness for which a defined cause is claimed. This is a claim of specificity. Does this test fail? It would fail if some patients reported symptoms that look like post-traumatic stress disorder but without a serious trauma event. If we call this serious anxiety, panics and depression rather than post-traumatic stress disorder, then some patients report this because of other life events that we might not initially identify as traumatic, if measured against our own experience. The life event is reported as distressing, but does not make the traumatic event list (whatever list we use). To express this more clearly, category B to H symptoms from the Diagnostic and Statistical Manual list may occur without the criterion A event.

We can say that traumatic events can cause post-traumatic stress disorder because the report or demonstration of a bad life event increases the probability or severity of post-traumatic stress disorder. However, if we discover that psychological disorder can be found without the narrative of bad life events, then the second test of specificity fails for two reasons. A specific relationship requires the trauma event to always cause post-traumatic stress disorder and the absence of the event to always mean no post-traumatic stress disorder. Not all trauma event victims get post-traumatic stress disorder. Examples were given above and these need to be explained. One explanation is that such people cannot recognize their distress because it is too distressing. However, this kind of repressed memory explanation suffers certain disadvantages, discussed elsewhere. It is dismissed here because a lack of evidence does not constitute evidence. Since bad life events do not always cause psychological illness, we should enquire why not and consider the implications of this.

Two examples follow. Patients were diagnosed with depression by standard psychiatric interview [8]. The interview enquired after bad life events. Of 103 subjects, 54 reported a trauma event serious enough to qualify for criterion A. These 54 subjects were assessed for the other post-traumatic symptoms and 42 (78%) qualified for post-traumatic stress disorder. Patients without a trauma event were asked if they had any fears or troubles that worried them. All other life events collected were divided between either not traumatic or equivocal between trauma and non-trauma. It was also decided if their symptoms qualified for post-traumatic stress disorder if there was a criterion A event. Thirty-six patients' life events were not traumatic, but 28 (78%) would have qualified for post-traumatic stress disorder. Thirteen had equivocal events, of whom 11 (85%) would have qualified for post-traumatic stress disorder. Therefore, of depression patients who lacked a criterion A event, the proportion with post-traumatic stress disorder equivalent symptoms was similar to the proportion of those who qualified for criterion A.

Military veterans attending a mental health service run by the United States Veterans Administration were assessed with a standard traumatic stress symptom questionnaire [9]. They were also asked to report their worst life event. These patients were divided up into those who met criterion A and those who did not. They were also asked to rate a list of symptoms on a zero to five distress scale. No differences were found on the questionnaire between criterion A positive and negative cases. Both groups were equally likely to qualify for post-traumatic stress disorder level symptoms. However, the criterion A patients were more likely to report core symptoms such as flashbacks.

Therefore, there are people with severe psychological disorder that is not called post-traumatic stress disorder because there is no agreed or obvious trauma event in their history. They have life events that they interpret as distressing. We could conclude that there is a psychological disorder, one route for which is signposted by a criterion A experience. However, there must be other routes. We could conclude that there is no logical necessity for trauma events to be a specific cause of post-traumatic stress disorder. Dose dependency shows trauma events can be a cause. Lack of specificity shows they do not have to be. There are discussions in relevant journals on the viability of criterion A [10, 11]. A more precise definition reduces the probability by 30% that victims of a trauma event are considered to have post-traumatic stress disorder [12].

One approach to this issue is to ask what we want a diagnosis for. The best reason is to decide the method of treatment. If we can avoid any objective judgement of trauma events and substitute the patient's subjective account of distressing images, then we do not have to worry about criterion A.

We can also neglect the idea of post-traumatic stress disorder. This conclusion creates a paradox. The illness is defined, presented and worked with as a pathology of subjective emotions, but such a report does not help us understand the cause, or at least, all the causes.

2.7 POST-TRAUMATIC STRAIN DISORDER

The history of post-traumatic stress disorder shows that the explanation varies between attributing all pathogenic influence to the trauma event or attributing the disorder to some interaction between the event and the patient's vulnerability [13]. Accepting this distinction is somewhat forced, I advocate the second explanation. Since most people, say 90%, do not get post-traumatic stress disorder or similar after a misfortune, then we are obliged to accept that the other 10% either have more than their fair share of bad life events or more than their fair share of vulnerability. We now consider a problem of definition, which leads into a problem of rhetoric.

If the definition of post-traumatic stress disorder includes stress, what can we say about this cause? In what sense is stress a causal agent? What is stress? The problem with this term is that it conflates cause with effect. The same word is used for both an external event and the internal reaction. It would seem the original reason for this is linguistic confusion. Hans Selye originated the use of stress in our context [14]. He was an Austrian physician who ended up in Montreal. Therefore, he was obliged to think in German, French and English. In a fortuitous discovery during research into female hormones in laboratory rats, Selye noticed a general response to any unfavourable stimulus. He subjected rats to various unpleasant substances by injection, or to extreme or life-threatening physical environments. Necropsy of these unfortunate rats showed a common physiological change (enlarged adrenal cortex; atrophy of thymus, spleen and lymph glands; and stomach lining ulcers). Selye postulated that this was a non-specific response to many pathogenic agents.

This is different from the specificity required to define a pathogenic agent as the cause of a specific illness. Selye originally named these internal changes 'general adaptation syndrome', but decided he needed a simpler name. He chose the word 'stress'. In physics and engineering, stress is the force acting on an area or object. The point is that 'stress' describes the external force, not the internal response of the object to the force. The internal response is called 'strain'. Selye reports that he chose the word stress because of its non-specific nature, as he understood it [15]. When he advocated the use of the word stress, his English was not sufficient to distinguish between stress and strain. In this way, external cause became confused with internal reaction, because stress was used for both. He also reports that the terms 'nervous stress' and 'strain' were then used by psychiatrists to describe the effects of life events. He wanted to avoid 'strain' so there was no implication of psychopathology. Here is the origin of our confusion. The current diagnosis of post-traumatic stress disorder implies a specificity that Selye rejected.

In some accounts of this problem, the word 'stressor' is used for the external trigger and 'stress' is used for the internal reaction; that is, strain as defined above. This seems redundant and confusing, given the distinction between stress and strain already exists. Another way is to distinguish between distress, a bad internal reaction, and eustress, a good internal reaction. References later in this book to a distress score using a 0 to 10 scale should really refer to a strain score.

It is reasonable to object to the conflation of stress and strain because the distinction is preserved in related subjects. For example, in ergonomics (industrial or work psychology), stress is external and strain is internal. Each is defined and measured differently [16]. The distinction is also retained in occupational medicine. For example, anxiety and depression in navy personnel can be called 'strain' [17].

Because the definition of post-traumatic stress disorder confuses the disorder with its cause, the patient's internal reaction (strain) is conflated with the external event (stress). This vitiates any ability we have to judge the strain independently of the stress. All stress is judged harmful. This confuses and subverts discussion of the effects of bad life events. If the cause is a morally engaging narrative, there is a risk that effect will be assumed. When the patient claims to be suffering from stress, we are forbidden, or at least discouraged, from enquiring if the stress has resulted in strain. If damage is assumed, then any stress is considered as harm and is, therefore, morally engaging. This may confuse how people think about their problems, or imagine them. It may explain why reports of the effect of difficult life events assume vulnerability, not resilience.

Veterans of difficult jobs, such as the military or police, might regard a claim of stress as sufficient cause to justify disability. Patients who claim stress as the whole illness may become angry, or consider themselves oppressed or unfairly treated if questioned on this [18]. Stress events undoubtedly exist in such occupations, such as the policeman who enters the barn to discover a suicide or the soldier first to the site of a suicide bombing. Such events can be reported with distress and require treatment. However, we should not relinquish the right to enquire what strain has occurred. This confusion has been observed before, but persists today [19,20].

Perhaps this failure to make the distinction will show up during treatment. A patient required serious surgery after a transport accident. He attended for assessment and agreed he had flashbacks to the accident. He remained calm. Since a patient who does not show obvious upset can still require treatment, he went forward to treatment. Two sessions of eye movement treatment failed to show any effect. He remained calm, while still reporting high distress scores. This happens sometimes and is difficult to explain. Perhaps this patient had been told by all around him he should have post-traumatic stress disorder, given his serious injuries, and had believed it himself, but did not have it.

This rhetorical misadventure might be the origin of confusion in the treatment of post-traumatic stress disorder patients. If one does not distinguish between external and internal events in assessment of the patient, then we will not find that strain can be less than the stress. This is sometimes referred to as the patient's resilience. If one cannot distinguish between stress and strain, then one will not believe that eye movements, or other methods of tapping on neurons, can reduce strain, particularly after a severe stress event. One might feel reluctant to clearly question patients about their bad life events in the manner advocated later. It might be difficult to accept that the patient's distress complex is limited to seven distress images, on average, as I shall later claim. Please notice I am obliged to refer to distress images and scores in this work, when strain images and scores might be better.

This abdication of enquiry might be the origin of the opinion that one is not allowed to contradict or question a victim, either self-declared or validated. It might be the origin of the opinion that all actions, comments or opinions that might cause distress, or be claimed to cause distress, should be forbidden. Such opinions invalidate any resilience or moral agency the victim might possess. There is a risk that the claim of post-traumatic stress disorder is based on an appeal to emotion instead of the logical basis that a good diagnosis would have. None of this is to dispute that some people who suffer bad life events get a psychological illness or disorder. This is a serious issue, with practical implications. Patients with post-traumatic stress disorder cost twice as much for hospital care compared to those without [21]. However, we might be better off calling it post-traumatic strain disorder.

Disagreement with the enterprise of psychiatric classification is still expressed, but I have never heard a good reason for this objection. The only reason I am aware of is that a psychiatric diagnosis has been used, in certain times and places, for political oppression [22]. Perhaps some objectors think this is true of our time and place. We should remember these victims and use diagnosis as liberation.

We should distinguish between disputing classification as an enterprise and disagreeing with the current achievements of that project. Classification will change and improve as knowledge grows, but this does not invalidate our current understanding. What do we want a diagnosis for? Like all forms of category and concept, we want to predict the future from the past. If a patient reports a certain symptom syndrome, can we help with a certain method? Perhaps a better diagnosis might be distress image syndrome, which would predict an improvement with eye movement desensitization.

3. WHAT IS REMEMBERED?

3.1 CLASSIFICATION OF MEMORY

The theory and practice of eye movement desensitization, as given here, requires some foundation in memory research. As we listen to the report of the patient, we need to understand what sort of memory is being reported. We may need to ask for, and explain, semantic memories. Not all trauma episodes are remembered or reported. In fact, most are not. This is mostly normal forgetting, but other reasons for memory lineations are listed. This does not require any dramatic explanation, such as 'repression'. In this chapter, I consider some relevant aspects of memory. If not all victims of bad life events end up with distressing memories, one reason may be that not all events, good, bad or neutral, are remembered.

For our purposes, memory classification can be mapped like this:

1. Short-term memory (working memory)
2. Long-term memory
   a) Procedural memory
   b) Declarative memory
      i. Semantic memory
      ii. Episodic memory
      iii. Autobiographical memory

Memory is initially divided into two parts:

Short-term memory

This is better called working memory. It has a limited capacity of around seven items, or chunks, of information. Overloading this limit may cause anxiety-based illness and is discussed later.

Long-term memory

This is further divided into two parts.

1. **Procedural memory**. This is memory for 'procedures'. These are actions that cannot be readily translated into words or those that no longer require such articulation after practice. Driving a car is procedural memory, unless one is a driving teacher. Procedural memory can be further subdivided, but we will not do that here.

2. **Declarative memory**. This is memory that needs to be translated into words, or 'declared'. Declarative memory can be divided into three further parts:

2a **Semantic memory.** This is memory for abstract facts and general knowledge. 'Semantic' means 'classified by meaning'. (For example: Heraklion is the largest city on Crete.)

2b **Episodic memory.** This is memory for personal events. Episodes are identified, or tagged, by time, place or source.

(For example: I visited Heraklion when I went to Crete.) For our purposes, time tags are the most important. If the same event is experienced repeatedly, it loses individual time tags and passes into semantic memory.

2c **Autobiographical memory**. Episodic memory is the preferred term here, but sometimes autobiographical memory is referred to. This is personal episodic memory. (For example: 'I remember we had lunch in the restaurant by the harbour, before we visited the Venetian fortress.')

3.2 EPISODIC AND SEMANTIC MEMORY

Semantic and episodic memory share some common parts of the brain, but also each can be shown to have unique activation sites [23]. A non-clinical example relates episodic memory to semantic. Respondents remembered how often they had signed cheques or used automatic telling machines [24]. They reported how they remembered these facts. The responses were validated against bank records. For small numbers of events, individual episodes were remembered. Episodic recall decreased rapidly after this small number increased. For one to two withdrawals, episodic recall was used for 88% of respondents. For three or more, this decreased to 21% and to 0% by ten episodes. Respondents used an estimation method. For example, such a strategy might be: If I wrote two cheques last week, I probably wrote six over three weeks. This is semantic memory knowledge of arithmetic.

Distinguishing between semantic and episodic distressing memories is required for our purposes. Many reported flashbacks are episodes and therefore episodic memories. However, distressing memories may be semantic. Some patients, such as domestic abuse victims, will have suffered multiple trauma events. They may report certain significant episodes that stand out, but the rest is semantic (for example: I remember my father abused me between the ages of 8 and 15). There might be a semantic memory of an abuse act, which was repeated until it lost its time tags. The individual episodes will be dissolved into a semantic memory. Semantic memories can be treated with eye movements in the same way as episodes. This can be used in abuse or assault cases. The patient is focused on the semantic memory of the repeated assault. The semantic memory may decompose into episodes, or require unpacking to make progress. It can also be decomposed into the face or voice of the assailant, because this would have been seen or heard on all occasions.

The episodic brain function may provide the ability to see oneself both in the past and in the future. The brain uses the past to model the future. Similar parts of the brain work to do this [25, 26]. Elsewhere, the importance of images of future catastrophes is discussed. These are called 'flashforwards'.

3.3 ARE ORDINARY THINGS REMEMBERED ACCURATELY?

Memory failures are a common experience. Here are eight reasons for non-clinical memory failure. The first six are taken from Schacter's list of seven reasons for memory failure [27]. The seventh on Schacter's list is the persistence of painful memories. Since this is the subject of this whole book, it is not included in this list. I have added two more reasons: memory illusions and infantile amnesia.

1. **Transience**

This means forgetting. Forgetting occurs rapidly after an episode, or after memorising the material for a test, for example. After that, the rate of forgetting decreases, assuming no rehearsal or use of the memory. As we all discover, this tendency increases as we age. Transience is a normal experience. The only surprising thing is that memory of bad life events can be transient.

2. **Absent-mindedness**

Here the information was not encoded to memory properly. This is as much attention failure as memory failure. For example, one puts down the house keys. A short time later, when one needs to leave in time to catch the bus to work, the keys cannot be located. Because the matter was not given sufficient attention, the key's location was not learned. The solution is to hold on to the keys for a few seconds and take a second look at the location, but one has to remember to do this.

3. **Bias**

Respondents tend to report memories that fit more with opinions of events or of themselves than an objective account may support. For example, depressed patients recall bad memories.

4. **Blocking**

Here the memory is encoded and the respondent has that sensation, but something prevents identification. This is known as the 'tip of the tongue' feeling. The most common type is name blocking. One meets and recognizes an acquaintance in the street, but cannot produce their name. Embarrassment ensues, which is doubled if both people block on the other's name, as once happened to the author. With names, the explanation is simple.

Most names probably described some characteristic of the person who originally required naming. As time goes by, other people inherit or acquire the name who do not share such ancestral characteristics. Also, with enough historical time, language has changed and the original meaning of the name might have become lost. The network of associations that locate this memory are lost.

5. **Misattribution**

An episode is reported, but the time or place label of origin that should tag it is lost or mistaken. The earliest type of misattribution described was called déjà vu. This is an illusion of familiarity about a current event, as if it has happened before. It has not, or not necessarily so, but it has lost a time tag identifying it as a current episode. Another type is source amnesia, where the respondent remembers a fact, but not where it was learned. Information might be reported from the wrong time or place, or from the wrong person or newspaper. It might be attributed to the wrong lifetime, causing fantasies about memories of past lives. A respondent may report being a queen in ancient Egypt, but have forgotten seeing a film about Queen Cleopatra [28].A respondent may also report information but not remember that it is a memory. This is cryptomnesia, discussed further by Baker [29].

6. Suggestibility

The circumstances of an inquiry may suggest a false answer to the person being questioned that is given to please the questioner. These circumstances are called the demand characteristics. It may that an interrogation leads to a false confession or witness identification.

7. Memory illusions

Sometimes a memory glitch may be an illusion, related to perceptual illusions [30]. Relevant here is 'telescoping', which I can report becomes common as one gets older. This is the feeling that an event happened more recently than it did. They seem closer in time, as if seen through a time telescope. Such episodes have acquired an illusory time tag. Flashbacks and distressing memories are telescoped.

8. Infantile amnesia

Autobiographical memories are not reported from the first two to three years of life [31]. After this, the proportion of memories gradually increases to about 20%, which seems to be the adult number. Patients may report abuse memories from this time. Such reports may require some careful discussion because such memories may not be veridical, but reconstructed from later information. Such reconstructed memories can still be eye movement desensitization targets.

3.4 ARE BAD THINGS ALWAYS REMEMBERED?

Bad events are not always remembered and there are examples of forgetting serious incidents. Violent episodes experienced by women in a Chicago public housing project were investigated [32]. Twenty-five women retrospectively reported trauma events, such as violence, rape or robbery, over the preceding 6 weeks, either personally or observed. They reported 132 incidents, biased to the more recent. The frequency of remembered trauma episodes per time interval was converted to incidents per year for comparison. For the preceding week, incidents were reported at 31 per year equivalent. For the preceding 1 week to 1 month, 14 incidents per year equivalent were reported. For the preceding 1 to 2 years, incidents were reported at only 0.4 per year. These were serious incidents; 16% involved deaths and violence was common. In the second phase, six of these women were interviewed prospectively, weekly over 10 weeks. The rate of trauma incidents reported then rose to 42 incidents per year.

Another difficult life event that can be forgotten is that of a mental illness episode. In New Zealand, the Dunedin Health and Development Study has been tracking a cohort of people since their birth in 1972 or 1973 [33]. A mental health assessment for common mental disorders happened at ages 18, 21, 26 and 32. This prospective prevalence data was compared with retrospective recall of illness episodes. About half the recorded episodes were recalled. For example, lifetime prevalence for anxiety was 49.5% compared with a retrospectively remembered 25% to 30%. The lifetime prevalence for panic was 6.5% compared with 3% to 4% remembered. The prevalence for depression was 41% compared with 16% to 19% remembered. This is a lot of episodes to lose.

In our third example, a cohort of young adults who were child sex abuse victims were tracked prospectively [34]. Court records from 1985 to 1987 and a previous research project validated the cases. There were 168 subjects in this follow-up. Of these, 142 (81%) reported the index case. Seventeen (9.1%) denied being involved. Seven (4.0%) reported other sexual abuse but not the event recorded. Two reported no memory of the abuse, but that they had been told about it by their parents. Seven did not answer the survey for various reasons. There were predictors of disclosure. Respondents were more likely to report if: (1) the abuse ended when they were over the age of 5, (2) it was more severe abuse or (3) if they had maternal support. In total, 19% could not report the index event.

There is a meta-analysis of 16 such reports where objective evidence was recorded through interviews both in childhood and in adulthood [35]. Reports of child abuse events, such as sexual, physical and emotional abuse, neglect, domestic violence, and other bad life events, was aggregated for children under the age of 18. This found 25,471 respondents with matched reports. This allowed comparing childhood reports to establish if the events were correctly reported in adulthood (prospective). The result was that 52% of respondents with childhood records did not report it in adulthood. Second, adult reports could be validated by childhood records (retrospective). The result was that 56% of adult reports could not be backed up by childhood records. Put simply, half the childhood records of abuse are not reported in adulthood and half the reports of childhood abuse by adults cannot be validated by childhood records. This warns us that asking a patient to list bad life events and previous health history, as will be advised later, may miss episodes.

3.5 REASONS FOR UNREPORTED DISTRESSING MEMORIES

Why whould bad life events not be reported? [36] Below is a list of reasons that must be excluded before other explanations need to be considered. The first six items are based on lists found in McNally [37] and Bower [38]. This list is added to the non-pathological reasons for memory failure listed above.

9. Psychological amnesia, which presents rare cases where a patient reports a loss of memory, often personal information. Such cases usually resolve with time.

10. Organic amnesia from biological or physical trauma causes. This might be concussion, drug use or other disease.

11. Choosing not to disclose for some reason such as embarrassment or shame. Domestic violence victims are more likely to tell a computer than interviewers [39]. In an internet study on two large samples of respondents, 81% and 61% had not reported something medically relevant to their doctor or nurse [40].The second sample was biased to older respondents. The top four reasons given were not wanting to be judged or lectured, not wanting to be told that their behaviour was harmful, embarrassment, and not wanting to be thought difficult.

12. Just not thinking about something for a long time.

13. Childhood sexual abuse victims may not recognize the

event as abusive until the gaining of adult wisdom, or finding a more honest public attitude to such matters. Victims of abuse by priests may not admit it to themselves or others if the priests have de facto immunity because that religion has acquired legal privileges in a particular jurisdiction. It was the legal situation of the Catholic Church when I was writing this chapter that inspired this observation [41]. No doubt there are other examples.

14. Failures of communication in the interview. The patient may not report because the question was not specifically asked. If the question was asked, the patient might just not have been thinking about the event at that moment.

15. Losing individual episodes of bad life events because of transfer to semantic memory.

16. A patient may identify a life event as bad, but not report it in interview because of a failure to identify this event as the cause of the current difficulties.

17. There is evidence for a memory illusion in which the patient reports remembering a bad life event, concluding it was previously hidden [42]. However, it was remembered previously but the patient had forgotten this previous remembering. For example, a patient remembered an abuse incident during eye movement treatment, reporting it as a new recollection. Her wife was present in the treatment session and reported that she had told her about this several years previously. One can develop this. The respondent may remember, forget, forget the remembering and remember forgetting. ('There was a period of my life when I did not know this.') There is a controversy concerning how bad

events are remembered or not remembered, which I will not pursue further than the section on repression below. Please consult other works for a fuller discussion of this problem. These difficulties are avoided if your method of psychological therapy does not require a veridical account.

3.6 ARE BAD EVENTS REPRESSED?

When bad life events are not reported, what are the reasons for this? The most likely explanations are those above. Another explanation sometimes still met with is 'repression'. Here is a recent definition of repression [43]:

> *Repression is a defensive strategy that keeps from consciousness unpleasant or unacceptable memories, emotions, desires or wishes. The concept involves the act of pushing down memories and restricting their access to awareness. A repressed memory is one that is forgotten from the subjective perspective of the person in whom the repression occurs.*

Psychoanalysts postulate that their patients suffer from reminisces. Therefore, if these distressing memories are identified and defused in some way, then the patient will recover. However, despite such treatment, some patients fail to recover. In this situation, to maintain that memories are the emotional pathogen, one is obliged to assert that further bad memories are still occult in some way. Psychoanalysts use the idea of repression to describe this. Older readers may recall that repression is associated with psychoanalysis and the theories of Sigmund Freud, an Austrian neurologist and psychiatrist whose ideas were popular in the 20th century. Psychoanalysis still seems to be taken seriously by some people, both as a therapy method and a source of metaphors.

I suspect that some people still believe that psychological therapy consists of the uncovering of hidden memories by an insightful therapist, and further, that this revelation is the mechanism of cure from emotional illness. Such insight is useful when it is achieved, but this cannot be relied on. In the definition above, the repressing person will push distressing memories away from awareness into the unconscious to avoid distress. Imagine a train stopped halfway out of a tunnel because the news from the first half of the train was bad enough to discourage the second half from coming out into the light. Perhaps this metaphor just elaborates the question rather than answers it.

There are problems with this claim. We cannot claim that the absence of evidence is evidence. How are we to test if a failure to report a memory is evidence for that memory? We know a distressing memory exists only when the patient reports it. However, once reported it is no longer repressed, or forgotten or not reported for any other reason. If repression disappears once we observe it, then it is removed from any possible rational study. If one imagines that therapy is investigating the patient for unconscious thoughts or memories, then one risks an accusation of some professional conceit. The therapist is claiming a privileged pathway into the patient's memory that no previous questioner has successfully negotiated. This is a claim of narrative privilege. By requiring the acquisition of hidden facts, the therapist completes the story. It is an overshoot of narrative determinism.

Another argument against the existence of such a memory mechanism is biological. Any animal that evolved a capacity to lose a memory of risk would not survive. Any human that repressed the memory of lions would be cat food. There are other objections. If we wish to take seriously that repression means real dangerous events become occult in some way, then we need to prove the existence of the founding event. In fact, this is difficult to do unless previous information is available. Stricter definitions tend to disappear the claim [36]. If it is argued that our first definition was too strict, then repression loses most explanatory power. It becomes no different from other reasons why episodes are not reported. If repression becomes a metaphor for remembering things with distress, the idea of repression will find wide application but little predictive power. If distress is the indicator, then such memories are identified retrospectively in therapy.

Perhaps this distress is acquired with hindsight. Eye movement desensitization patients may report new memories and other information during treatment, sometimes with distress. This may include the report of physical sensations. A rape victim may report a vaginal pain sensation. An assault victim who suffered attempted strangulation may report breathing difficulties and the sensation of hands constricting the throat. The rare case may react physically and verbally to this remembering. This can be dramatic, and dealing with such distress is considered in Chapter 8. A dramatic presentation does not validate the memory or require repression or any other special mechanism of memory as explanation.

Any previous absence of such reports could be governed by one of the reasons listed above. Also, decomposing a semantic memory into episodes is not evidence of repression. The correct question is: do we need to accord that act of remembering any privileges, such as calling it repressed? No, we do not. There is no need to accord that new memory any narrative, explanatory or curative privileges, because we are doing eye movement desensitization. I am always surprised when psychoanalysis is taken seriously, given how systematically it has been trashed in anti-Freud books [44]. In my opinion, psychoanalysis and Freudian theory are little more than a hall of mirrors best avoided. There is much published on repression and similar things, such as dissociative amnesia, psychogenic amnesia, and its dangerous descendant, false memory syndrome. It is not the purpose of this work to enter this arena. The reason I wish to (briefly) take this corner and make this case here is that I will later try to persuade you that the number of bad memories or images we need to treat with eye movement therapy is limited. Accepting any credibility of repressed memory would reduce this position to the untestable.

3.7 SCRIPT

What to say to the patient:

Sometimes when the same bad thing happens repeatedly, people do not have individual memories of each time. They all become combined together into one big bad memory of (trauma event). Please imagine this repeated bad event, at all the different times it happened, are stacked on top of each other in your brain. You are looking down through them. What do you see? What they have in common shows up strongly. The time tags will be different and fainter. Is this what it feels like to you? It may be that you have one big bad memory, but you may also remember the worst time as a separate event. We may need to treat both.

4. IMAGES AND BAD THOUGHTS

4.1 INTRODUCTION

Eye movement desensitization is indicated for all patients reporting toxic imagery. The indication is not limited to post-traumatic stress disorder, which is a movable diagnosis often used to describe any distress. Most reports of distressing life events, and some other disorders or illnesses, can be reduced to targets that can be treated by eye movement desensitization. This includes some that did not previously indicate psychological treatment. These possibles are listed in Chapter 7.

Issues with assessment need consideration since the account of eye movement desensitization given here depends on accurate assessment and measurement. Measurement is considered in the next chapter. Advice on full psychiatric assessment or on determining risk is not given here. Also omitted are problems of differential diagnosis, such as distinguishing between flashbacks, hallucinations or pseudo-hallucinations. Assessment for eye movement desensitization is similar to assessment for cognitive behavioural therapy, but is more specific. For example, a patient receiving prolonged exposure might be asked to focus on the car accident memory. For comparison, this is the breakdown during eye movement desensitization treatment of a road traffic accident case into nine flashbacks:

1. The sudden appearance of the car that hit the patient's car.
2. A 'flashforward', in which the driver imagines his wife injured in the accident. (His wife was in the car, but not injured.)
3. The feeling of suddenly braking and being jerked forward.
4. The silence after the impact.
5. The feeling of being trapped in the damaged car.
6. The police telling him to exit the car.
7. His wife screaming (a sound flashback).
8. Looking at the crushed car, having got out of the car.
9. The accident as a whole event.

There might be a series of sensory images, such as the below for a generic rape victim. If there was more than one assault, these flashbacks are semantic, not episodic.

1. The whole rape episode
2. Vaginal pain sensation
3. The weight of the rapist's body on the victim
4. The face of the rapist
5. The voice of the rapist
6. The body smell of the rapist
7. A flashforward to anxiety in certain locations where the assailant may be encountered

Each of these flashbacks may be broken down into the eye movement desensitization triad and distress score. Not all are required. The right flashback is the one that reduces with eye movements:

1. The image
2. The negative cognition
3. The physical feeling
4. The distress score

We require a brief diversion to consider the history of and alternatives to the word 'flashback'. In our context, the word is of recent origin, since about 1980 [45]. This word is not that respectable and does not deserve any imputation of truth. The word may have been borrowed from the cinema, where flashbacks are a common narrative device. Originally, it was used for intrusive memories and panics due to drug-induced hallucinations, not real events. Another problem is that the patient may deny having flashbacks if the distress memories and images can be controlled. Perhaps the most generic term is 'eye movement desensitization targets', but this does not sound very psychotherapeutic. Sometimes the informal word 'trigger' can be used. Another word used in some reports is 'hotspot', which I suspect means the same. However, it is difficult to find another word that is as convenient as 'flashback'. Eye movement desensitization is discussed here as aimed at flashbacks, but other types of target are considered later.

The therapist may have to deconstruct the inquiry for patients who need extra coaching. For example, some good questions to identify flashbacks are:

1. Do you have clear memories of the event (or other source of distress), like a film in your head?
2. Are these memories distressing in some way, perhaps when you are reminded of them?
3. What was the worst part? Most scary? Most disgusting? The part that makes you feel sick? That brings the pain back?
4. When did you realize the bad thing was going to happen?
5. When did you think you were going to die?
6. Do you remember when you lost control?
7. When was the worst pain?
8. Do you have clear pictures in your head about the thing that scares or distresses you?
9. Can you see the face of the person who committed the assault or bad life event? How tense does it make you feel?
10. In your mind's ear, can you hear the voice of the person who said the bad things?
11. In your mind's nose, can you smell the body smell of the person who did the bad thing?

4.2 NOTES FOR INTERVIEW

This is a summary of my usual eye movement desensitization interview, as a list of what is important. This is intended as guidance for beginners, and those therapists who believe asking chronic distress patients about what distresses them is too distressing for the patient. Experienced therapists will have their own interview routines. Eye movement desensitization is explained to the patient at the end of the interview, when need is established. Some patients will not discuss their painful business until they know the benefit. The explanation should then happen first. If in doubt that the patient is a candidate, let the patient decide. This is a version of the psychotherapy manoeuvre of making the dilemma explicit. Eye movement therapy is not a secret and candidates will often know about the procedure. I do not worry if the patient is ready for the procedure. The patient is ready if they attend the appointment. The patient who is not ready will refuse consent, dissent or fail to attend. In my clinic, the patient will often attend to request this treatment.

The interview style recommended here is clinical and business-like. If this is explained first thing, the patient will generally say that style is preferred. On occasion, I will say to a distressed patient during assessment or treatment, 'Are you still OK with my way of asking questions?' They always agree and we can continue. A statement at the beginning that one will be clinical, business-like and pushy is a rhetorical device to define the boundary between what I want them to do and the patient 's right to informed consent.

At the beginning of the appointment, check the patient knows who the therapist is and why the patient is there. State that the appointment will last one hour. The patient should not be embarrassed by showing distress or anger, since that can be part of the interview. The interview is in four parts:
1. The patient's description of the problem.
2. Background demographic information.
3. Specific assessment of the patient's problem, leading to assessment and measurement.
4. Have we missed anything?

The patient's description of the problem

Ask the patient what the problem is. This allows the patient to say whatever is on their mind or to unload immediate causes of distress. If the patient talks for more than about 15 minutes of the hour, move on to the next section. The patient can be interrupted with an explanation that the interview must keep to the agenda. Three problems may arise. First, some patients' need to explain their life, and issues may be so great that they are best left to do that. The formal interview can be put off to the second appointment. This is as much about courtesy as clinical judgement. Second, the patient may be so distressed that the interview cannot proceed. In this case, interrupt and explain that this distress will be discussed later, but in a specific way that will be easier. Then proceed to the next section. Last, the patient may choose not to start like that or produce only a few sentences. Proceed to the next section.

Background demographic information

1. Family background

Age, place of birth, parents' status, father's job (and mother's), status of siblings and relations with family. Any family health problems and bereavements. Any marriages or equivalent relationships. Why did marriages end? Are there children? If there are broken marriages, or other relationships, with children, ask about contact. Also, briefly visit their housing and financial status. A burden of debt must be acknowledged, even if there is no way to help with this.

2. Education and employment

Age of leaving school or other education, qualifications, employment history, current or last employment, job satisfaction, reasons for unemployment. Disability or medical retirement status. If military, enquire after combat status ('Did you see any shooting?').

3. Health history

Any relevant medical problems, disability, operations or diseases. Write a list of medical problems. Is the patient in pain? Is the patient under any medical care or needing a diagnosis? Assume nothing. A letter of referral can fail to record a close call with cancer several years previously. Patients will often identify depression on this list. Write a list of bad life events. Is there any current active psychiatric, psychological, counselling, or religious help? Any current diagnosis or treatment may require negotiation with other clinicians or may contraindicate eye movement desensitization. Sexual history and sexuality may have to be enquired after. Sexual history is relevant for sexual assault victims, but the enquiry may be redundant and distressing for a patient with chronic pain. In a sexual health clinic, explicit enquiry about sexuality may not be required if the patient is referred with that information.

4. Anything missed?

Ask if there is anything that has been missed out of the interview that the patient thinks important or needs to be said. This is with the deliberate exception of not assessing all bad life events in the first interview but only using one as the example.

This information has three functions:

1. These questions should be part of any good clinical interview.
2. Asking some mundane questions allows a distressed patient to calm down and get used to the situation.
3. It is likely that this report of life history and circumstances will identify distress triggers for further questions.

All bad life events the patient remembers, or wishes to report at that time, should be listed in the first interview. I attended a case review where the patient was discovered to be a child abuse victim after several treatment appointments for an armed robbery. This was presented as a problem for treatment, which it is. However, such narrative surprises can be avoided by asking straight questions in the first interview. Patients may be distressed when they discuss this list, but that is the point. That distress is the problem requiring help. We should not be embarrassed about distressing a chronic distress patient because we know eye movement desensitization reduces distress. However, do not assess the whole list of bad life events to find the high distress score that indicates eye movement desensitization. Usually, only one flashback or distress memory needs to be assessed to qualify. Ask the patient to describe the most distressing. If not ready to do this, ask for the flashback the patient is able to deploy today. This may be episodic or semantic. ('Think of all the times your husband assaulted you. Does it feel like one big bad memory?') When a qualifying distress is found, the assessment is finished. Perhaps not all the bad life events on the list will require treatment, and treatment may be needed on images that are not bad life events.

Specific assessment of the patient's problem

The rest of the chapter considers three components of assessment. These are the image, the negative cognitions and any bad physical feelings. In other methods of psychological therapy, the meaning of each would be the therapeutic material. This is not required in eye movement desensitization. Assessment for eye movement therapy locates that place in the memory network where the flashback is located. The image, bad thoughts and bad feelings are a grid reference to a memory location. The distinction between the three is, to some extent, an artefact of assessment. Eye movement desensitization therapy can be launched if only one or two out of three are present. Reasons for this are discussed below.

4.3 IMAGES

Flashbacks and other eye movement desensitization targets are a subset of mental images. Images are the pictures, or the internal sensation of such, that our brains use to show us information. Images are only pathological when distressing, confusing or inhibiting in any way. Traumatic imagery is not just visual. One military veteran patient reported finding a truck full of the burned remains of enemy soldiers in the desert during a patrol. The truck had been hit by a missile. *We could smell it a kilometre downwind as we approached it. I can still smell it today, after 20 years.* Eye movement desensitization patients will report images of smell, sound, pain or physical impact [46]. One solution to problems in treatment is to dissect out the different sensory modalities and treat each. This is discussed later.

There is evidence that images are models of the original perception. The word 'model' is sometimes used to mean explanation, but I do not mean that here. This model is something in the brain that can be shown to share some characteristics of the original perception. Several examples follow.

1. Jacobson's original work

In 1932, Jacobson observed that the relevant muscles reacted when subjects imagined using them [47]. For example, electrical signals were detected in the right arm when the subject imagined lifting their right arm. Signals could also be detected in the eye muscles corresponding to imagined images.

The example given is a subject asked to imagine the Eiffel Tower from bottom to top. The eye muscles signalled a vertical movement as this image was imagined. This reaction decreased with relaxation. This example is historically significant, because the systematic desensitization procedure was based on this observation. Systematic desensitization is the attempt to reduce the arousal caused by an image by relaxing the muscles. Eye movements seem to do this better. The reports of Antrobus et al., from 1964 and 1965, are similar [48,49]. Eye movements were observed to be highest when the subject was asked to imagine active images such as a tennis match or when asked to suppress an image of a particular life event.

2. The pendulum

In a similar finding, subjects asked to imagine a pendulum showed side to side eye movements as if following the real movement [50].

3. Smell

Olfactory imagery can cause people to sniff. Subjects instructed to imagine a smell image will sniff more than baseline sniffing and more than when instructed to imagine a visual image. When asked to imagine a pleasant smell, subjects will sniff more than when asked to imagine a bad smell [51].

4. Imagining exercise

There is interesting work on motor, or movement, images. In one report, heart rate and oxygen use when using a treadmill for three minutes were determined for three speeds [52]. Heart rate and oxygen rate increased with speed. In the imaginary equivalent, the subjects were put in three equivalent situations, but with the treadmill stopped. A tape recording of progressively faster treadmill sounds was played to encourage them. When imagining this effort, heart rate and oxygen use also increased. The increase was only about a quarter compared with actual exercise. It was dose dependent. Faster imaginary treadmill speeds caused a larger physiological response.

If we instruct a patient to imagine a flashback or other anxiety trigger, we are asking them to create a mental model of the original event. This will have similar effects to those detected in this laboratory work. By using this as an eye movement desensitization target, we are aiming at a model of the original event. It is a model in the sense that the visual image is 'seen' in the visual cortex (at the back of the head in the first instance). I find it useful to imagine that the primary visual cortex is a screen onto which the image is projected. This cinema metaphor is a simplification of a complex reality, but gets us started. The image might be of a real external object or an imagined image in a clinical or laboratory task. Brain imaging shows the relationship is topological so that the centre of the external object will activate the centre of the visual cortex. Other parts of the object stand in a geometrically equivalent relationship in the visual cortex.

After the primary visual cortex, other visual maps exist. A total of thirteen maps have been detected in the brain [53]. When we instruct our patients to pay attention to a bad visual image, we are asking them to use these parts of the brain. This is a minimum, since other parts of the brain must also engage.

Does post-traumatic stress disorder activate the visual cortex? To some extent it does. Brain imaging of post-traumatic stress disorder was performed on patients with symptom provocation. That is, the patients listened to a recoding of their bad life event story while in the scanner. The scan showed increased activation in various parts of the brain [54].

This included the mid-occipital region, which is the site of the visual cortex. Other areas concerned with autobiographical memory and self-concept also lit up. Experiencing distressing memories is more complex than just visual system activation. However, there are issues with allocating a psychological event to one, or a few, brain locations, to be considered in a later chapter.

There are two kinds of visual images corresponding to two points of view. **Field images** are those where people see things from their own point of view, as if reliving the experience. They are sometimes called first-person images. **Observer images** are where people observe themselves in the scene, as if in a film. During eye movement treatment, patients will report either field or observer memories. The distinction is not required in assessment. The change observed in treatment corresponds to a change from field to observer view, if the patient started in the field view. Then there is an enlargement of the observer perspective. That change is often the first sign of progress. Patients are often surprised and it may be necessary to stop the procedure to discuss this change.

4.4 IMAGES HAVE BEEN USED BEFORE

Other psychological therapy methods use images. Here is an example of a systematic desensitization hierarchy for a medical phobia from the 1982 edition of *The Practice of Behavior Therapy* by Joseph Wolpe, the originator of behaviour therapy [55]. The numbers are subjective units of a distress score on a 0 to 100 scale.

1. The sight of physical deformity (90)
2. Someone in pain (50 to 90, depending on pain level)
3. The sight of bleeding (70)
4. The sight of somebody seriously ill (60)
5. Automobile accidents (50)
6. Nurses in uniform (40)

7. Wheelchairs (30)
8. Hospitals (20)
9. Ambulances (10)

This is clearly a hierarchy of images. We recall that in systematic desensitization, the patient is taught to relax and then asked to imagine their way up this ladder of disturbance. Each stage begins when the preceding stage has reached a low score.

Images are used in cognitive therapy. Aaron Beck, the originator of cognitive therapy, described these pathological images in 1970 [56]. Beck includes images as cognitions and refers to these as 'fantasies'. This might be a flashback, but also might be a 'flashforward' to an imagined catastrophe in the future. There are also symbolic fantasies, if that is the best term. For example, a patient angry with his mother sees her distorted into a fierce animal. Beck and Emery's 1985 manual leads on the determination of bad thoughts, but considers images in two ways [57]. Images can also be the primary pathology and therapeutic target. Methods are given to directly change the images.

Two are:
1. De-catastrophizing or rescripting. This means determining the associated bad thoughts and deconstructing the errors with the patient.
2. Repetition or prolonged exposure. The patient is asked to deliberately repeat and describe the fantasy image. When this happens, the distressing image changes towards reality. Beck observed that if the patient was instructed to repeat

the image, it became more rational. If the patient repeated it on their own, without instruction, it stayed irrational.

4.5 BAD THOUGHTS

The negative cognitions requested for eye movement desensitization are similar to, and may be identical to, the negative automatic thoughts requested in cognitive therapy. Beck's original procedure required tapping into the narrative self-talk people hold with themselves. The internal dialogue of distressed patients contains an excess of negative automatic thoughts. Some of these will be wrong.

If the internal dialogue of a terminal cancer patient is, 'It's terrible and it's not going to get better', this will be correct enough. Usually, the bad thoughts of a depressed patient will include those that are wrong as a matter of fact, or at least could be disputed. One method of cognitive therapy is teaching identification of such bad thoughts and the antithesis when the bad thoughts are unjustified. Such negative automatic thoughts often have a catastrophizing theme.

Negative cognitions in eye movement desensitization are excused the role that negative automatic thoughts have in cognitive therapy. In cognitive therapy, the bad thoughts are an issue because the premise is that they cause the emotional illness. We could say they have narrative power. Since cognitive therapy is effective, this premise is valid. In an eye movement desensitization assessment, patients may report neatly connected bad thoughts, but will more likely report the raw emotion ('I am scared'), paired with an image or sensation. This label is used to navigate to the correct place in the memory network and draw the patient's attention to that place. It is not about determining a link in the chain of causal logic that can be broken because it is not logical. It is convenient if such causal bad thoughts can be found, but this is not required in the eye movement procedure. Later, a theoretical distinction is made between two classes of psychological therapy: rhetorical and procedural. Cognitive therapy is rhetorical, meaning the words are the agent of change.

4.6 BAD EMOTIONS

Put simply, there are two opinions on emotions. We can think of them as the hardware and software theories. In the first, certain emotions as we know them are represented as such in the brain at some neurological level. These emotions are hard-wired in as such. Alternatively, emotions are found in linguistic codes, current and past experiences or cultural convention. Emotions are labels we use to describe body states and sensations that are not specific to named emotions or brain locations. They are software programmed on top of more basic sensations of the body that can be reduced to either good or bad.

The idea that emotions are brain hardware is called basic emotion theory. Basic emotions are more 'biological' and the atoms from which compound emotions are built [58,59]. The criteria for basic emotions and the number considered basic can vary, but we will use this list:

Good basic emotions: Joy, surprise.
Bad basic emotions: Distress, anger, fear, disgust.

For example, disgust is on the basic emotion list and makes a good eye movement desensitization target. It can be understood as a basic biological emotion because it protects us from infection risk and other disease vectors. Disgust is a factor in many presentations, not just those involving bodily triggers, and should always be watched for [60,61].

Other emotions that are reported to us are secondary to the basic emotions. For example, I would include anxiety, as distinct from fear, as secondary. Fear should be distinguished from anxiety, since fear may be justified and perhaps not treatable to zero by eye movement desensitization. Expressions of phobia and depression are secondary. Other expressions of distress can also be understood in this way. For example, the 'I feel dirty' thought reported by sexual assault victims could be fear, disgust, shame or guilt (if self-blame is reported). Definitions of emotions can be fuzzy. Are hunger and thirst emotions or something else, such as primary biological drives? Eye movement desensitization patients will become tired in treatment and there is an argument that fatigue is an emotion [62].

The second theory of emotions is more helpful to our purpose. It can be found in Barrett's useful book *How Emotions are Made* [63]. In this book, the theory of basic emotions is criticized as follows: The argument that some emotions are basic is circular. Basic emotions are detected and identified by subjects who are shown pictures of actors posing those emotions. However, such methods contain contextual clues to the emotion. In other words, there are clues to the correct answer. If the context is changed, or the clues reduced, the accuracy in identifying basic emotions decreases. In the original basic emotion research, subjects were shown a picture of the target emotion, let us say fear, and asked to choose which it was from a list of basic emotions. In this test, there will be a strong preference for fear. If the clues are reduced by showing the face without the list, then fear is chosen much less often.

If the question is asked, 'What word best describes what is going on in this person's head?' so there is no clue that an emotion is required, identification of fear decreases further. If there is less context and fewer clues, the ability to identify the emotion is reduced. Therefore, there is no innate ability to recognize emotion. Recognition can be shown to depend on the subject's context, emotional vocabulary, previous experience and cultural history. If identification of emotions can be changed, by changing the context, then basic emotions can no longer be considered as basic. This account of emotions is called constructionist. Constructed on what basis? They are constructed on internal body sensations, which are referred to as affect or core affect. This is a perception of the physiological body state and our need for energy.

This body perception is a sense called interoception (formed from 'internal' plus 'reception'). It includes such things as heart rate and blood pressure. This signal is combined with previous experience and other sources of information to predict the body's energy needs. Affect has two dimensions. First, is it pleasant or unpleasant? That is, feeling good or bad?

Bad emotions are constructed on a bad core affect and good emotions on a good core affect. Perhaps one way of thinking about this is that we now have only two basic emotions or motivations that might be labelled as emotions or something else. The second dimension is how distressed, aroused, agitated or switched on you are.

We can write three conclusions here. First, perhaps the arousal level of a bad core affect is what we measure with the distress scale (see the next chapter). Bad core affect might be the same as, or the cause of, strain, as discussed in Chapter 2. Second, when using the distress scale, I advise switching emotional labels to find the highest score. This finds the best label to locate the highest core affect. Third, an assessment for eye movement desensitization is divided into image, cognitions and physical feelings. However, there may not be any useful distinction between emotion, cognitions and physical feelings. If we can run these three together into the same category of core affect label, we do not need all three in an assessment, or at least we can start without the full set.

4.7 PHYSICAL FEELINGS

As declared above, questions about physical feelings may be redundant. Treatment targets are usually defined well enough with image, bad thought and distress scores. If emotions are labels for core affect and interoceptive cues, then perhaps further discussion might be redundant. However, as we proceed, the patient may report different physical feelings not yet qualified for an emotional or cognitive label. Physical sensations may include nausea, tension, pain or 'heavy feelings' in various parts of the body. This can include medical symptoms or, more precisely, physical sensation images of interoceptive signals of medical origin. Here is the route to using eye movement desensitization with medical patients. Medical symptoms that cannot be diagnosed for a medical treatment may be called 'medically unexplained symptoms'. Here we can call such reports physical sensation images and ask for the score, not a diagnosis.

These descriptions can be idiosyncratic, but can be used in three ways. Firstly, if the patient has difficulty finding an emotion label, ask for the physical location of the bad feeling. 'Can you feel a lump of (bad feeling) inside you? Please point to it and give it a score.' Secondly, a cognitive label such as 'It was my fault I was assaulted' in a sexual or physical assault victim may be attached to a physical feeling. Ask, 'Can you feel the lump in your chest that means it was your fault?' Discussion of attribution of blame is required, but we should desensitize the self-blame feeling to zero first. Third, the body scan is recommended at the end of eye movement desensitization to determine if all physical sensations are finished. The various indications of distress may not decrease in synchrony. Each needs to be checked.

The expression of symptoms will vary. In a medical clinic, this may cause a problem with detecting distress. Busy doctors or nurses may only find distress if the signs are obvious. Chronic distress that is not shown may go undetected, unless by explicit measurement. The next chapter deals with this.

5. THE MEASUREMENT OF DISTRESS

5.1 HOW TO MEASURE DISTRESS

Assessment for eye movement desensitization requires the measurement of subjective sensation. This might be anxiety, tension, pain or whatever label is reported and gives the highest score. The label might be an emotion, a bad thought or a physical feeling that has not yet found such a label.

Verbal descriptions are required, but do not determine the correct treatment target or show direction of change. A simple zero-to-ten scale serves our purpose. Zero is no internal sensation. Ten is the worst, either experienced or imagined. The patient is asked to score the sensation now, in the appointment. It may be necessary to emphasize the required score is not their memory of the trauma event from when it happened, but as experienced now. The patient may define that distress score of ten by that event, but the score required is here and now, during assessment or treatment. This scoring is inherited from earlier behaviour therapy methods, such as systematic desensitization. This quantitative assessment is an essential premise of the eye movement desensitization procedure advocated here. How are numbers reported by the patient real numbers? We cannot count them, like a pile of beans. The answer is that numbers do not have to be 'countable' to be useful numbers.

I use the term 'subjective unit of distress' in this book. This can be introduced as a 'bad feelings scale', naming the relevant bad feeling, elsewhere referred to as a distress scale or a strain scale. A high distress score identifies the flashback. Changing the label on a flashback can result in a higher distress score. For example, a flashback to a panic attack may score low when labelled with the bad thought 'I am going to die from a heart attack'. If the bad thought is changed to 'I am embarrassed to panic when people are watching me', then the embarrassment score may be high. The therapist should always find the highest number, like a hiker should always climb the highest hill for the best view.

5.2 NUMBER SCALES

There are different sorts of number scale and we should enquire what kind of scale the distress scale may be. This classification of measurement is taken from Stevens' system, originally published in 1946 [64]. This system has been debated, criticized and expanded by mathematical psychologists, but is useful here. There are four types of number scale: nominal, ordinal, interval and ratio. The fourth type, ratio scale, is divided into two further types.

Nominal scale
In a nominal scale, the numbers are used as a convenient name, not as a measure. For example, the number 119 bus. This type of scale is not relevant here.

Ordinal scale
In an ordinal scale, the numbers are ranked in order, but we do not know how much space is between them. Assume the series 1, 2, 3, 4, 5, 6, 7... is ordinal. We can then assert that 1 is smaller than 6, but we do not know if 1 to 3 is the same distance as 4 to 6. To take a non-psychology example, in 1822, geologist Friedrich Moh devised a mineral hardness scale. Each rock on this list can scratch any below it, so it is harder. However, this will not be directly related to whatever property of rocks makes them harder. It merely ranks hardness [65]. Most psychological and symptom scales are ordinal. The symptom lists for post-traumatic stress disorder and panic in Chapter 1 are effectively ordinal scales. If we measure our patients with a questionnaire as they go through treatment, which is the best policy, we are using ordinal scales. Ordinal scales are adequate for informing clinical decisions, such as 'Is treatment finished or do we continue?'

Interval scale

In an interval scale, numbers have equal intervals, but there is no number zero. The scale is anchored to the real world at one point in some arbitrary way. There is no such thing as zero intelligence, but there is an intelligence quotient (IQ) score that most people can achieve. The most common score is the mean and is allocated a value of 100. The scale is then calibrated either side of the mean in a normal distribution curve. A second example is the calendar year scale. There is no year zero, other than by convention or retrospective belief in the arrival of a prophet. Interval scales are not relevant here.

Ratio scale

These are numbers as we generally know them. They have a real zero and there are equal distances between each number. Again, consider the series 1, 2, 3, 4, 5, 6, 7… as ratio numbers. Not only is 1 smaller than 6, but we have enough information to know that 1 to 3 is the same distance as 4 to 6. A ratio scale is defined by equal ratios. For example, the ratio $6/3 = 8/4$. For our purposes, there are two kinds of ratio scale:

Linear scale

This is the scale we generally know and use. The numbers are evenly distributed, left to right, along an imaginary number line. Please look at your ruler for an example of this. Our arithmetical and measurement systems are generally linear.

Logarithmic scale

The nervous system is a logarithmic system. In a log scale, the higher numbers are compressed towards the high end, according to some mathematical protocol. Instead of the 1,

2, 3, 4, 5... of the linear scale, we would see, in the simplest example, 1, 10, 100, 1000, 10,000, 100,000... (= 10^0, 10^1, 10^2, 10^3, 10^4, 10^5...). One way to understand a logarithmic scale is to think about money. Money has an objective amount, which is how much we own. It also has another value, which we call subjective utility.

Utility means how much we value additional money, given our current objective holdings. The more we own, the more we require to be impressed by that further amount. If I own £100, then I will be happy to acquire another £10. If I own £1,000, then I will be less impressed by acquiring another £10. If I own £100,000, then I would not notice the next £10, but would be impressed by acquiring £1,000. The higher I get on the money scale, the larger the difference I require to make me notice that difference. The scale compresses the higher we go up it. Ten pounds means less the more money it is compared with.

5.3 A SENSE OF NUMBER

Please do this for me. On the desk in front of you (or wherever you are) you will see an object such as a pencil. Please pick it up, look at it and put it down again. This is easy, unless you are suffering from some neurological misfortune. You looked at the pencil, measured the distance to it automatically and calibrated your arm movement to intercept it. Measurement is an innate property of the nervous system. Perhaps we could call it another sense. Any organism that cannot measure will not be able to navigate its environment, locate the necessities of life or avoid the lions and snakes. We exploit this for clinical benefit. Eye movement desensitization taps into this ability and cannot be done without it.

The anatomical basis for measurement can be found in the brain [66]. A meta-analysis of 93 brain imaging reports mapped the brain sites for three number tasks. First, that signalled for tasks of estimation of quantity, but without using numbers. Second, for magnitudes such as physical size, again without numbers. Third, for numbers as symbols and numbers of objects, such as dots. These three measurement tasks showed both activation sites that combined the three measurement types, but also unique sites for each.

Let us initially simplify this a stage by saying there are two number systems in the human brain [67,68]. They are the approximate magnitude system and the exact number system. The exact system is a linear system that tracks small numbers of objects by assigning markers to them. This is restricted to about four to six items. This is probably equivalent to visual attention or working memory. Above that limit, the markers become symbolic numbers and then it is based on language and arithmetical education.

Brain scans of humans show neurons that detect numbers are arranged topographically in the right parietal cortex [69]. There are bands of cells tuned to one to seven. Smaller numbers have more space on the surface of the brain and larger numbers have less space. This fits with the idea that larger numbers are more difficult to detect and discriminate.

Neurons tuned to numbers can also be detected by recording from electrodes placed in neurons during brain surgery where the patient is asked to use numbers in a calculation [70]. Two groups of neurons were detected that activated with either numbers as symbols (5) or non-symbolic numbers, shown by a number of dots (for example: • • • • •). Neurons only showed one sort of number, not both. The number range tested was one to five, with five being the most common.

Neurons that respond to a number are optimally tuned to that number but respond less to the numbers before and after that peak number. If we imagine that brain number neurons are shown a number, say 5, the neuron tuned to peak at 5 will fire at their maximum. The 5-neurons will fire progressively less to 4 or 6. This gives us an approximate system. The approximate system is a mental number line. It is logarithmic, or similar. This mental number line has the property that discrimination between two numbers is easier the more space between them, and that discrimination is more difficult higher up the scale.

Which number system are we using when we ask for a distress score? We are probably using the approximate magnitude system because we are asking the patient to rate an internal subjective sensation with no external number as reference. However, asking for the number must require the number system.

5.4 VALIDATION OF SUBJECTIVE MEASURING

Validation means we can show that a subjective number scale correlates with and therefore measures something interesting in the real world.

1. Comparison with standard questionnaires

Sixty-one patients were treated with eye movement desensitization for post-traumatic stress disorder, depression or anxiety over an average of five sessions [71]. Subjective units of distress scores at different stages of treatment showed reasonable correlation with standard questionnaires, for impact of events, anxiety and depression. 'Reasonable' here means significant at around 0.4 and 0.6, which is an acceptable correlation value.

2. Distress thermometer for cancer patients

The subjective units of distress scale is used for cancer patients as the distress thermometer. It was validated by comparing the distress score with previously validated questionnaires and finding a good statistical correlation. Since questionnaires have to be validated when translated into different languages and the distress thermometer is used in many health services, there is much research [72]. Two examples follow. Distress scores, questionnaire scores and life problem lists were collected from 380 patients attending five cancer clinics in the United States [73]. The average distress score was 3 to 4. Distress scores showed a good statistical relation with the previously validated questionnaires. In a similar report, data was collected from 123 patients within 30 days of diagnosis [74]. The average score was again 3 to 4. The same good statistical relation was found with the questionnaires. These comparisons show that the best distress score threshold for distinguishing between 'not distressed' and 'distressed' was 3 to 4. Let us say 3 and remember that score for our own patients. In the method chapter, I advocate distress scores should always be zeroed, but 3 or below is good enough when that is not achieved.

3. **Subjective height**

Subjective estimates of height match real heights [75]. Altogether, 25 members of a university psychology department used psychological scaling to estimate the height of the other 24, relative to their own height as a comparison. The psychological measures showed a correlation of 0.98 with the actual height. This is good. If the relation were perfect the correlation would have been 1.0.

4. **Aircraft in the air**

To take an example from ergonomics, air traffic controllers can validly estimate their work strain caused by controlling aircraft [76]. A subjective measure of work strain, reported by the controllers, was correlated with the number of aircraft each was responsible for (at $r = 0.97$, which is high). The controllers' heart rates also correlated with the number of aircraft.

5.5 MEASUREMENT IS GOOD

Why does the type of scale matter to eye movement desensitization? First, what sort of scale is the distress scale? The distress scale may have a real zero, because the patient is told zero is zero distress. Zero distress is clearly observable and that is a qualification for a ratio scale. But there is no objective external number for a subjective sensation. Therefore, we must consider the distress scale as a non-numerical magnitude system which is probably logarithmic. This means the distress scale will be less precise at high values. Or at least, the lower the distress score goes, the more discriminating it will be.

However, the score can only be reported using numbers. The human number ability and arithmetic system must be based on the approximate, or logarithmic, number system, which is an emergent property of the nervous system. The symbolic numbers we use are an interpretation of this innate number line, using the numbers taught to us in school [77]. The patient will use the number system to report the distress value. The report will often be something like 'it is between 5 and 6' or 'it is a high 3'. This sounds like the patient is looking at a magnitude line and using a number to communicate their position on it.

We now make the conservative assumption that this is no longer a ratio scale. We cannot be sure that a decrease of 10 to 7 is the same desensitization distance as 6 to 3. This is not a problem, because we do not need to know this. If we assume that the distress scale is ordinal, that is all the information we need. An ordinal measure has the properties we need to make a clinical decision. We just need to decide to either continue eye movements or stop. We only need to know which direction to go in.

If the reader doubts these are genuine usable numbers, please remember mathematics uses infinitesimals and the square roots of complex numbers. Measurement is a separate chapter from assessment, because it is key to good eye movement desensitization. It is necessary to assert that subjective sensations can be measured, but not in the same way as counting beans. This is fortunate since the Subjective Unit of Distress (or strain) is required to discover the treatment target, which might not be some significant episode of the trauma story. The highest score may be a semantic memory, not an episode that fits the narrative.

This change of score measures a titration of eye movements against distress. All distress images should be reduced to zero or other acceptable low score. The report and measurement of distress, or strain, is homologous with physical pain. A medical patient will be asked to score pain on a zero to ten scale. This is done because physical pain is not always obvious. There is no dial or control panel in the middle of a patient's forehead that shows the pain and measures it. Emotional pain, or distress or strain, is the same. Often the only sign in a cool and competent patient will be a high distress score. This is why all flashbacks need to be reassessed, either at the beginning of each session or at some point in the treatment sequence. The only exceptions are those that will not zero for some good reason, which is considered later in this book.

This distress titration defines the units of treatment; that is, the flashback or other toxic image. I shall later try to persuade the reader that there is a limit of seven toxic images, on average, per patient. This claim will hold only if we can define the images. Distress measurement defines the images. It is our friend and should be treated as such. Furthermore, distress scaling is the patient's friend. A patient's distress is not increased if they are asked to measure that distress. I suspect that for most patients, being asked to measure distress is the first step to understanding that it can be controlled and reduced.

5.6 WHAT TO SAY TO THE PATIENT

Commonly, patients with medical problems will know the zero-to-ten physical pain scale and understand how to apply this to emotional pain. Here is a suitable script:

One of the problems with eye movement desensitization is that it can be difficult to find the words to describe the change. This is a problem everybody has. It does not mean you have turned stupid or lost your words. There are two solutions. You can measure your feelings about this bad memory on a 0 to 10 scale. This is the same method a nurse uses on the ward when they ask you to rate your pain on a 0 to 10 scale. This is like an imaginary ruler, where 0 is 'I am OK' and 10 means you feel as bad as you can, whatever bad feeling is relevant.

Don't worry how you do this. Most people can do it. This is easier than trying to find the words to describe a strange experience. Have I explained this OK?

Sometimes people have difficulties with calling a number, or feel it does not work for them. If this happens, don't worry because there is a second way to see how you are doing. Please choose one of the five alternatives. Do you feel better, worse, the same, different, or not sure yet?

6. METHOD

6.1 SUMMARY

For our purposes here and to a first approximation, eye movement desensitization is prolonged mental image exposure accelerated by eye movements so that it is not prolonged. The image is defined and measured more precisely and more often. Other forms of sensory stimulation have the same effect.

The patient holds the flashback in attention while performing a repeated eye-tracking task with the therapist's instruction and assistance. Eye movements are performed in sets of about 25. After about 10 to 15 sets (in a simple case), the patient reports that the flashback progressively turns into normal factual memory. This is not just the visual, but also associated images such as sound, smell, physical contact or pain. There is no correspondence between sense used for treatment and image sense being treated. Visual eye movements reduce sound images and auditory on/off stimulation reduces visual images. As this happens, the associated distress, anxiety and negative automatic thoughts decrease and disappear. New information or memories may be reported. Patients will report new information as images, sometimes with distress and physical reactions. Eye movement desensitization is best understood as a titration. Eye movements are administered until the distress score reaches zero or some low plateau. In my experience, the total dose per patient is about 100 sets of eye movements about seven to ten flashbacks. This is an average figure with clear exceptions, usually involving panic or physical reactions. This chapter describes eye movement desensitization in a minimalist and almost algorithmic way. All distress images and triggers must be treated. The generic rape victim will report assault flashbacks, but also child family issues and social anxiety. We do this because we can, because this will increase her or his resilience to future risk and because a clean working memory is a life asset. Because we treat semantic memories as well as episodes, this is a limited number of targets. Can you use eye movement desensitization on different things? Read the next chapter. What happens when there is a problem? Read Chapter 8.

6.2 INTRODUCTION

This chapter is a protocol for eye movement desensitization, which originated in notes made in 1991, before formal training was available. It is taken from Shapiro's original reports [78,79]. The canonical account can be found in the third edition of Shapiro's manual [80].

This chapter disputes about half of that taught on the approved courses for eye movement desensitization and reprocessing. Notably, certain things are omitted or only done if need arises. The omissions are listed in the last section (6.7). This chapter does not substitute for training, which should be taken when the opportunity arises. At least the Level One course should be taken. The new eye movement therapist should ask for advice and supervision. Some patients are beginner's cases and some are not.

To get the full benefit of eye movement desensitization, it is important to distinguish between this and other psychotherapeutic methods or models. Eye movement desensitization is a powerful and effective procedure when it is correctly performed on the right patient. Combining it with other methods is a waste of time for both the therapist and the patient.

The therapist should know how to deal with any possible crisis. For example, a patient's reaction can cause the need to vomit. One patient's nausea was so strong, she ran to the toilet to be sick. On her return, she reported feeling much better because she had 'vomited the rapist out of her system'. Make sure the patient knows where the facilities are for such an occasion. Chronic pain patients must be able to move as necessary to ease the pain. Asthma patients must bring their inhalers. The therapist should know what to do in a medical emergency. A patient with undiagnosed medical problems reported increasing cardiac pain during eye movement treatment. It became plain this was not a pain flashback or physical response to the treatment. Since the author works in a medical hospital, the emergency doctor was called, who admitted him for observation. No doubt the protocol in psychiatric or psychotherapeutic clinics is to call an ambulance. The therapist should be clear about emergency procedure.

6.3 USE OF AIDS AND TOOLS

In the original method, therapists used their fingers as the guide to move the patient's eyes. I recommend that two sorts of artificial aids can be employed in eye movement desensitization. This does not include the light bar, which I have never used and regard as rather elaborate for the task. I also think it breaks a connection between therapist and patient. A stick with a target at one end can be used to guide eye movements [81]. Other methods of sensory stimulation have the same result. The auditory method is achieved with sounds in alternate ears. The tactile method uses taps, or vibrations, on the patient's hands. This is best done using the right equipment, which can be used to deliver either alternating auditory stimuli through standard headphones or a vibration stimulus to the hand. This employs two plastic tactile probes. These are plastic oval shapes about the size of a coin, containing a rotating device that causes vibration. Both the auditory and tactile stimuli are driven from the same 'signal box' [82], which is a battery-powered signal generator. There are two reasons to acquire such kit.

A career of repeated arm movements over a large radius must be avoided. It would be painful and result in some kind of injury. The choice of sensory modalities allowed by the signal box allows treatment of patients with eye problems or sensory disability.

A patient lost most of his sight during a military mission. He later became sufficiently hearing disabled to refuse auditory stimulation. I spent several sessions tapping on his hands with pens before purchasing a signal box and using the tactile probes. This made the procedure easier and more dignified for everybody concerned.

Patients do not have problems with such tools and often prefer to use them. Some people do not like moving their eyes and will choose auditory stimulation. Others prefer to keep their eyes closed to concentrate. An alternative method can be used when eye movements become tiring for the patient but we need to finish a bad flashback. There may be a problem if the patient has been assaulted with a stick or device similar to what the therapist proposes using. In my experience, two patients have objected to the stick on these grounds.

6.4 FIRST APPOINTMENT

The assessment and measurement described in Chapters 4 and 5 happen now. The patient is briefed and informed consent obtained. The patient's understanding of the procedure is required for success. It may be necessary to explain that eye movement desensitization is not hypnosis. The method is described and any particular problems identified. The therapist should demonstrate the eye-tracking task by moving their hand from side to side in front of their own visual field and tracking with their eyes. If a stick or signal box is to be used, introduce and demonstrate these. Explain that painful and personal memories will be dealt with in a business-like and clinical manner. Most patients respond positively to this. I usually reach the briefing in the first one-hour appointment.

The briefing should be adapted to each patient and any individual issues discussed. For example, is the patient still at risk in any way? If nightmares or sleep paralysis have been detected, discuss it with the patient and state that it will be included in the treatment (see Chapter 7). What are the circumstances under which eye movement desensitization will happen? No doubt in the same place as the first appointment, but any problems with this should be identified and discussed. The therapist and the patient should sit so that their eye levels are equal. The patient might like to have somebody else present, such as a spouse, partner, friend or chaperone. This can be helpful if that significant other can later discuss events. Most patients choose not to have somebody else present, perhaps because of embarrassment or possible distress.

Another issue concerns the treatment of sexual trauma victims by therapists of the opposite sex. The (male) author routinely deals with female rape and abuse cases without a chaperone. This is in the context of routine sexual health clinics on the other side of the treatment room door. Female patients presumably take the situation into account when consenting.

The author's chaperone rules are; under 16, patient request or therapist request if some issue aroused concern.

When the patient consents, book the treatment appointments. The author books three, each one hour long. Appointments are for eye movement desensitization and any other therapeutic business inside this time should be restricted. The rest of this chapter describes the procedure for these appointments. It is in two parts: (1) how to treat individual flashbacks and (2) how to deal with the series of flashbacks and finish.

6.5 TREATMENT OF INDIVIDUAL FLASHBACKS

Reminder and starting the session

At the beginning of the first treatment session, briefly remind the patient of the procedure and establish a stop signal:

I will ask you to focus on the flashback and move your eyes in sets of 25 eye movements. It should change. This may take you by surprise and perhaps confuse you at first. If you have a problem, stop me and ask a question. If I think you are having a problem, I will tell you the answer. If you wish to stop suddenly for any reason, say so or raise your hand.

Assessing and recording the flashback

To establish the first flashback, elicit and record the three parts of the flashback: (1) the image, (2) the cognition, emotion label or self-statement, and (3) the physical feelings. Flashbacks can go back 50 or 60 years. The flashback may not be to the event initially reported. The report may not be visual, but can be a smell, sound, physical sensation or pain. For example, a patient reported that she heard, 30 years ago, the abuser downstairs opening the door to the house. In such a case, ask: 'Does it feel like you can hear this sound again, in you mind's ear, now we are talking about it?' The flashback may be semantic rather than episodic. That is a combined report of similar events. If reporting is a problem, ask the patient to describe the most difficult part of the memory, and identify the image and label from this. Summarize back until the label is recognized by the patient as correct and specific to the image. Certain cognitions and emotions can cause problems. Embarrassment is embarrassing to admit. Feelings of guilt may be hidden. Anger may cause a fear of committing violence. Identify and locate the physical symptoms, if any. These will probably be physical anxiety symptoms, but the patient may describe something else. Ask the patient to rate the flashback on the distress scale. Most patients will understand how to do this, but some never take to scaling distress or cannot apparently do so.

If the patient becomes distressed, there is no need to finish assessing the flashback. Because they are distressed, it is likely they are focused. When the patient is still distressed but ready, proceed with eye movements until the distress is reduced. One example of this that rape victim who can be started simply by requesting them to focus on the worst part of the rape. Eye movement desensitization requires constant assessment and measurement. The distress image can be reassessed at any time in the procedure. If the distress does not reduce, there is a problem, discussed in Chapter 8.

If several flashbacks are identified, start with the highest-scoring and work down to low-scoring flashbacks. Such high-scoring flashbacks may include panic or strong anxiety attacks, or strong physical responses. This rule can be expressed as follows:

We will start with the worst flashback if you can, because that probably makes it easier in the long run. However, if you do not wish to do this, then choose where you want to start.

If dealing with a sexual or physical assault, either single episodes or a series merged into a semantic memory, it is necessary to say something like this:

To begin, I want you to focus on the rape event as a whole thing and we will try to get rid of it as a whole thing. If we are lucky, this will work. We may get stuck and have to break it down into smaller chunks. In particular, you may get back a sensation or pain in your vagina (or other assault location). If this happens, tell me, because we need to get rid of this as fast as possible.

It does not matter if a flashback is not fully assessed for image, cognitions and physical feelings. As discussed in Chapter 4, it is likely these are all possible labels for interoceptive signals from below the neck. We can merge them into the same category. This is another reminder that eye movement desensitization is not a narrative therapy. The correct eye movement target is that which reduces distress with eye movements.

The visual tracking cue

Ask the patient to concentrate on the flashback. Put your

fingers, or stick, in the start position at eye level, in the centre of the patient's visual field. If a stick cannot be used, find some way of resting the elbow, on a desk or chair back, for example. Use two fingers, or the hand, since one finger might be interpreted as aggression. Ask the patient to nod when ready and to look at the stick, then to track the stick visually. When the patient nods, move the top of the stick from side to side or rotate it across their visual field, about 25 times. This is the set of eye movements, which is the basic unit of eye movement treatment. One count is both a left movement and a right movement, so that the stick returns to the start position.

As I recall, in my original training the original instructions specify 12 to 24 eye movements, about twice per second, at least 100 centimetres from the face, the distance travelled by each being about 30 or 40 centimetres. In my opinion, this is rather fast. Adjust the eye movements to the patient's comfort and experience with eye movements. It probably does not matter exactly how fast the eye movements are, but it does matter that the eyes do travel. Eye movements can be in different directions, such as up and down, diagonal or circular, to reduce fatigue. Continued difficulties with eye movements indicate another method of sensory stimulation or a more general problem with eye movement desensitization.

The set of eye movements
The therapist can decrease the number of eye movements if the patient reports difficulty or increase them to speed through a distressing stage. Shorter sets give more opportunity to check that the flashback is still focused. Distress may not provide

sufficient evidence for good focus. The patient may need to be reminded for each set which flashback of a distressing story is the currently chosen target. A third option is that the patient decides when the set should finish. This is helpful when issues of control are important. Some patients do not focus well until some time into a set. A fourth option is to do a series of sets of 25 without a reassessment of each. The patient is reminded and refocused briefly only between each series of sets. If the distress reduces, then the focused image must be correct and does not require reassessing between sets. An experienced patient will report any issues without prompting.

The flashback will change

In the original account, the patient was told to take a deep breath and blank out the flashback. Warn the patient that this might prove difficult at first, but will get easier. The function of the deep breath and the blankout appears to be to control possible upset. This may be necessary at first, but distress can be better dealt with by decomposition as described in Chapter 8. After a few seconds and when the patient seems ready, ask for recall of the flashback, to report other symptoms and to score the distress. Expect the visual image reported to degrade in some way and become progressively difficult to recall. Flashbacks in other sensory modalities will also change in an analogous way. The cognition and emotions will change from bad to at least neutral and perhaps to positive. The distress will decrease. Qualitative changes may occur. For example, anxiety may change to anger. Any new bad thoughts or more positive insight thoughts can be reflected back to the patient.

The distress score will tend to zero, or another stable low value, which should at least be below four. Patients can be taken by surprise by the speed of the change and may have to be reassured that this can happen. For each set, note the set number, the distress value and enough of what the patient says to remind them of it if necessary. For example: 'Set 8; Image less clear, I remember people helped, my chest feels less tight. S = 4 or 5.' The capital 'S' stands for the distress or strain scale number. Recording all the details may be unnecessary while the patient is improving. However, enough must be noted to remind the patient later of the flashback. For each set, reductions of one or two distress points are usual, but reduction of more may be seen. Progress can be slower. Four or five sets may be required for one or two points. The report of other changes is monitored. Such changes can happen without distress reduction and this is progress if the decrease happens later. This is the reprocessing part of eye movement desensitization and reprocessing.

A small proportion of patients have difficulty with distress scoring and progress must be monitored by other changes. Two suitable questions are:

1. Has the flashback changed in any way, or not?
2. Is it better, worse, the same, different, or are you not sure yet?

There may not be a change in the first three or four sets. It can take this long to start the process. It may be necessary to reassure the patient that this is normal. No change after four sets indicates a problem. In the initial stages, it is most likely that the flashback needs to be defined more carefully or decomposed into smaller targets (see Chapter 8). When distress is decreased, the patient may have to be warned that it will take progressively longer to focus the flashback. Pessimistic patients may fear that they are doing something wrong. Reassure them that this is the result, not a problem. In the later stages, patients may look puzzled and confused when questioned between sets. It may help to explain that if it feels like the questions are becoming irrelevant, this is a sign of progress. They feel irrelevant because they are becoming irrelevant. This advice may be required:

Sometimes people say they can focus on the flashback or watch the stick but not do both at the same time. Which is right? Simple answer: do what feels right at the time. It will work either way.

The flashback usually diminishes as described, but other changes may be reported. Anecdotally (i.e. it is my impression that) different kinds of changes can be reported as follows:

1. Distancing: the flashback recedes as described in the briefing.
2. Time distancing: the flashback retreats away in time. The memory telescoping illusion decreases.
3. Doughnut: there is a loss of focus starting from the periphery and encroaching into the centre.
4. Face and eyes: this is a subset of 'doughnut' where the face and then the eyes of a character in the flashback disappear last.
5. Reverse jigsaw puzzle: the flashback breaks up into pieces, which disappear one by one.
6. On/off: the flashback switches on and off.
7. Just the furniture. Sometimes the dangerous part of the

image will go away, leaving the furniture, literally or metaphorically.

8. Cinema. Patients will often use a cinema metaphor to describe the changes. For example, 'It feels like a film I saw' or 'It feels like the people are just acting'.

9. Colour change: the image changes from colour to black and white.

10. Echoes. Sound flashbacks become like echoes.

11. Optimists. Sometimes patients describe improvements that did not happen in the real story. For example, the rain stops and the sun comes out in a flashback of a road traffic accident, when in fact the rain continued and it was getting dark. A child abuse victim may say 'I can see myself fighting back, even though I was only eight'.

12. Does not happen. Sometimes the image does not go away at all, but is desensitized satisfactorily. Some people do not lose their images.

These descriptions may be useful. Sometimes patients appear not to make progress when the experienced eye movement therapist thinks they should. On such occasions, a careful enquiry such as 'Perhaps it is going fuzzy round the edges?' may be productive. One problem here is that the therapist might be cueing the patient about what is expected. However, the briefing should not have left any mystery. Such an inquiry may be needed to detect the first signs of change in a difficult case, to see if the procedure is running as it should. Any response that is fake or just offered to please the therapist will be revealed by subsequent lack of progress.

Fixing the flashback

This task is systematically repeated until the flashback and bad emotions, cognitions and physical feelings have either disappeared or changed to neutral. The distress will go to zero or some other low score. In my first audit database, the mode number of sets required is six and the mean is fifteen. The distribution of required sets is positively skewed. This means usually some six to ten sets are needed, but be prepared to go the distance to finish difficult, panicky or complicated flashbacks that cannot otherwise be decomposed. A large physiological component may slow progress. If the patient shows signs of this, explain the problem and continue carefully. Be prepared to decompose the target down into the sensations. The sensations are just interoceptive signals not yet labelled with an emotion.

The different parts of the flashback may not change in synchrony, especially towards the end of the process. For example, if the patient reports any residual physical feelings or tension, then focus on these symptoms. This is the body scan. The patient can be asked if the flashback is finished or if another set is needed.

Advising the patient

During treatment, issues may appear that require discussion or advice. It is best to avoid this. There is no point discussing an issue based on a bad thought that will change with the next few sets of eye movements. If it does not change, discuss it after all eye movement sets have been completed. Such issues should be considered separately, preferably after the treatment. Note the issues to return to later.

Eye movement desensitization may be exhausting and difficult for the patient. In this case, announce the end point of the session when it is clear from treatment progress. Finish around 40 sets.

6.6 TREATMENT OF SUBSEQUENT FLASHBACKS

The next flashback
If the first flashback is treated without problem, one of two things should happen. It will tend to zero, as considered above, or the patient will report another flashback. When a new flashback is reported, reassess and treat until complete. Then return to the first flashback, reassess and continue. Alternatively, note the second flashback, finish the first, then go to the second, flashback. It is possible to deal with two, three or even four flashbacks per session, if there is no problem.

Subsequent appointments
On the second and subsequent appointments, reassess each flashback collected and recorded in the notes. The patient is asked if it is impossible, difficult or easy to recall the flashback, to give a distress score and to report anything else important. If reactivation of a flashback is reported, then further eye movement desensitization is required. If the patient reports reactivated flashbacks or other symptoms over several appointments, then there is still exposure to the trauma, another anxiety trigger, unreported trauma memories or panics between sessions. Consistent failure indicates another

problem, such as factitious disorder, personality disorder, dishonesty or self-deception.

Ask the patient to identify any further flashbacks. Usually, a series of flashbacks is collected and dealt with systematically. Unless the patient prefers otherwise, always start the second or subsequent sessions with the highest-scoring flashback. Progressively take flashbacks off the list from the highest to the lowest distress scores. Deal with all reported flashbacks or distress triggers over whatever number of sessions are required. In the author's audits, this is an average of seven or eight flashbacks in an average of three sessions. A session contains around 40 sets of eye movements.

All reported distress images must be treated, not just those from the initial report. The following phenomenon may be observed. Treating high-scoring flashbacks may reduce the score on untreated lower-scoring flashbacks. For example, two flashbacks score nine and seven. The nine-score flashback is treated to zero. Re-scoring the second then shows a decrease to maybe 5 or so. Presumably the extent to which this happens shows that working memory capacity is cleared by removing the high-scoring images (Chapter 9), or that the the two flashbacks are associated or overlapping in the patient's neural network (Chapter 10).

Finishing the series

Eye movement treatment is complete when the series of flashbacks has disappeared or degraded in some way, related cognitions are neutral or positive, and the physical symptoms have finished. At this point, the distress should equal zero or some other low stable score. There are two methods to check if treatment is finished for one or a series of flashbacks, at any point:

1. Read back the flashback from the notes and reassess the patient.
2. Ask the patient to think of the incident as a whole and reassess any anxiety or distress shown. 'Think of the whole accident.'

Expected changes

Treatment is continued as long as distress images are reported and it is finished when all reported images have been desensitized and remain so for one follow-up appointment. There should also be improvements in any key behavioural test or general behaviour and distress symptoms. Assess and discuss these changes in the patient's life. Sometimes these will be specific to one flashback and fast. For example, a woman who was assaulted in the shower became able to shower comfortably and without panic. Sometimes behavioural improvements will be slower, more generalized and more difficult to articulate, and will only happen when treatment is complete. Other signs, such as recovery of sleep or sense of humour, can show. Some patients will just say something like 'I feel lighter' or 'I don't think about the bad things anymore'. Eye movement desensitization eliminates psychological symptoms specifically, even if the patient is sick, and even if that sickness is terminal, for example, cancer.

The presence of other psychiatric or medical problems can mask the effect of eye movement treatment. An assessment of improvement may have to allow for such problems. If the patient is depressed, there may not be any immediate improvement. For example, eye movement treatment will help an adult patient who presents with depression caused by childhood abuse. However, such patients may accumulate other reasons for depression in a lifetime of bad decisions. Such a patient may not be further helped by eye movement treatment. The patient may require another psychological therapy, or perhaps cannot be helped further. One patient successfully completed treatment, but the difficult circumstances of his marital break-up prevented any benefit. He remained depressed. The detection of such problems does not contraindicate eye movement treatment, since the therapist should never be pessimistic on the patient's behalf.

Handing control back

Because eye movement treatment is controlling and prescriptive to begin with, find ways of handing control back to the patient. When the eye movement treatment is working satisfactorily, the patient will take control back. To encourage this, ask for information and guidance from the patient. For example:

1. Ask what the next flashback is.
2. Reflect the flashback back to the patient and ask if this has been understood correctly.
3. Ask if the flashback is finished, rather than assessing it directly. 'Is that one zapped, or does it need another set?'

6.7 NOT INCLUDED IN THIS METHOD

Certain parts of the eye movement desensitization and reprocessing procedure are deprecated here.

1.The safe-place procedure is declared redundant since it represents an abdication from treatment. Since eye movement desensitization reduces distress in the treatment session, any increase in distress, or failure to reduce it, is a problem to solve in that context by a change in procedure. If the safe place or alternative methods of distress control are taught before eye movement desensitization, then there is no advantage gained from using eye movement desensitization.

2. No cognitive interleave is used. See discussion in Chapter 8.

3.The positive cognitions assessment is declared redundant. In the original procedure, patients were asked for a positive statement for each flashback that would be valid if it were not distressing. The truth value of the positive statement was rated on a one to seven Validity of Cognition scale. For example, a patient might be required to imagine she could cope with the effects of the rape. How true is that on a validity score of zero out of seven? The zero score means she did not believe she could recover from the rape. Having elicited the positive thought, the therapist will ask the patient to focus on it in the latter part of treatment on each flashback. Eye movements will then increase the positive beliefs in a similar way to how they decrease the negative beliefs. There is not necessarily any image or physical feeling reported at this stage.

I stopped using the positive cognitions procedure at an early stage. In one instance, both the patient and myself became confused by the attempt to elicit a positive statement immediately after arousing the patient's bad feelings. At this time, the patient was distressed and a sudden inquiry about what positive thoughts they might have in an ideal world seemed neither fair nor necessary. Further confusion was caused by the change from the zero to ten distress scale to the zero to seven validity scale. This omission did not seem to do any harm, and seemed unnecessary if all flashbacks were treated. When this procedure was omitted and the series of distress images was treated as described above, then healthier cognitions were reported without any encouragement.

There is a similar procedure called resource installation. I have never tried this, because I see no need to do it. My understanding is based on a reading of the protocol in Shapiro [80]. The resources required are positive emotions, images and self-opinions. The patient is questioned to establish them, asked to focus on them and to score positive emotions. Short sets of eye movements are then used to increase the positive emotions.

If I understand this correctly, both the positive cognition procedure and resource installation imply that positive cognitions and emotions can be increased by eye movements. I find this puzzling, since my understanding is that eye movement decreases therapy bad emotions and it seems unlikely that eye movement can both reduce bad effect and increase good effect.

We also need to note that this needs to be contrasted with those protocols that advise decreasing positive effect with eye movement therapy (for example, in addiction treatment).

The claim that positive cognitions and effect can be increased with eye movements is at least an anomaly, and unhelpful in my attempt to explain the eye movement effect in later chapters. There is laboratory evidence that shows that eye movements decrease positive emotions, not increase them. In my opinion, the use of resource development installation should be stopped [83].

The idea of installing good thoughts as a resource attributes some causal role to those good thoughts or emotions. I suspect this is part of the narrative explanation I am trying to persuade the reader to part company with in this book. In Chapter 11, we will call this cognitive or emotional determinism and discuss it further. In Chapter 9, I attempt to explain the benefits of eye movement therapy to unloading an overloaded working memory. The resource that eye movement desensitization installs is an unloaded, cleaner working memory.

6.8 DEBRIEFING

Debriefing and some discussion is required after the first, and perhaps subsequent, treatment sessions. The following points should be made after the first session and repeated if necessary:

1. The patient will feel tired and this shows the treatment has had some effect. Some people report headaches afterwards. It is just a headache. Take your usual tablet.

2. The speed of eye movement therapy may be confusing. The speed of treatment does not mean the patient imagined their problem.
3. New bad memories may sometimes appear between sessions. These are the next things to treat.
4. The patient should not drive a car or operate other machinery for 30 minutes after treatment. A colleague in treatment should not resume any clinical responsibility for 30 minutes. Nothing terrible has ever happened in that time. It is just a precaution.

7. DIFFERENT TREATMENT TARGETS

7.1 INTRODUCTION

Considered here are different types of flashback or distress images, other eye movement targets or sources of such targets. Any of these targets can be treated as described in Chapter 6 and the problem solved as described in Chapter 8. They will appear in series with any conventional flashbacks of a distressing life event.

7.2 REPORT OF NEW INFORMATION

In any psychological therapy, the patient may report new information. This may be new memories or new conclusions. This is generally considered a good thing. Patients in eye movement therapy will also do this, sometimes with increased distress or the report of physical sensations. This should not be taken as evidence of an inadequate first interview, but evidence that the procedure is working. Assessment for eye movement desensitization, as described here, does not require the collection of every flashback before treatment starts. Neutral, pleasant or even amusing information may be remembered. However, for some patients, new and distressing information is reported. It is usually a new component from an already identified trauma event. Occasionally it is a whole new event. Patients may report distressing flashforwards to events that have not happened. This new report with distress may be seen in about one-third of patients [84]. The briefing should warn about this possibility, which the patient should accept before consent. The patient may report non-visual flashbacks, such as the pain of sexual or physical assault, of an accident injury or of medical treatment. This is distressing for the patient, and the therapist should provide support during the acute phase.

Do not stop the eye movement therapy.

Reassess this as a pain flashback. If the pain location is non-sexual, request 'Please point to the pain'. Then continue. 'How much does the pain hurt on the 0 to 10 scale? Please focus on the pain and we will carry on, when you are ready.' Pain that appears with eye movements will decrease with eye movements, short of medical crisis.

A particular example is the rape patient who reports the pain of forced sexual penetration. Adult victims of childhood abuse may recall the sensations of a male abuser's ejaculation in their face. It is necessary to ask the patient to focus on these explicit trigger sensations to accomplish the mission. Avoiding these difficult issues does not help the patient. It defines the central part of the trauma memory and must be dealt with. Such risks must be identified for patients, who must accept the circumstances under which it might happen. Any specific reason for missing memories may be discussed in the briefing.

The rare case may react physically and verbally to this remembering ('Get him off me!'). The therapist should remain calm and talk the patient through this crisis. Although the policy in this situation is to continue treatment, this may not be possible, especially towards the end of the appointment time. This makes it an unclosed session.

Such reports have the following properties, in my experience. There are exceptions to these guidelines but this combination of events can be used as a guide:

1. This missing piece of the report may contain the physical contact with the patient.
2. The report can happen fast, often in the first session after five or six sets of eye movements on a particular flashback. Remembering can happen in subsequent sessions or between appointments. The end of session debriefing should warn about this possibility.
3. Patients who remember in this way usually do so only once, occasionally twice.
4. The new report will be a flashback that contains sensory information and be a specific part of reported events, not general allegations. Usually, recollection is both limited

and conclusive. It does not begin a series of revelations, but finishes them.

5. Recollections are not limited to childhood abuse. All types of trauma events can be reported this way. The patient can report a revelation of a possible future event, or flashforward, with equal distress as remembering a past event.

6. The distress must be controlled by the eye movement procedure. Recollection under eye movement therapy is a good indication, if handled correctly, not bad. The correct way is to continue treatment until the distress is reduced as far as is possible. The incorrect way is to regard the new revelation as therapeutic narrative in itself and stop treatment.

A new recollection may be preceded by an increase in distress. Investigate and assess the new memory and continue the treatment. The procedure will control the patient's distress. It is best to continue until that memory is desensitized, but this may not be possible if this happens at the end of a session.

If the new flashback is very distressing or is blocked, decompose it as discussed in Chapter 8. A revelation that happens at high distress should be treated. A remembering at low distress may indicate a stop to allow the patient to think things through. Focusing on physical symptoms may encourage this process. There is advice to avoid physical symptoms in the first session, but this is difficult to do with the direct style of treatment advocated in this book. Therapists with a background in traditional psychotherapy should not regard any insight gained by a recollection as curative in itself. The new report of a central trauma memory can be a difficult problem, but also a step forward. A missing piece of the story does not predict distressing recollection. Real or apparent memory gaps can also be caused by the issues discussed in Chapter 3.

7.3 SEMANTIC AND EPISODIC

Declarative memories – that is, those that can be spoken – can be either episodic or semantic. A semantic memory is a repeated episodic memory that has lost it's time identification, because it is not stored by time but by meaning. Semantic memories can be treated as the whole target. The patient can be focused on a semantic memory, formed from repeated similar trauma events and for that to desensitize as a whole thing. A patient with a 10-year history of repeated sexual and physical assaults by her ex-husband was treated in two sessions. We worked through six semantic memories of the assaults, which included pain and sensation as separate targets. Semantic memories may decompose into episodic memories, giving the illusion of memory recovery. Semantic memories that get stuck may require decomposition into episodes: 'Do you remember the worst assault from…?'

7.4 FLASHFORWARDS

Flashforwards are images of some anticipated disaster. Such targets do not seem to be less distressing for being acts of the imagination. Five examples are:

1. A claustrophobic patient reported a terrifying flashforward of being buried alive trapped in a coffin.
2. A flying phobic reported a flashforward of a plane ditched in the sea. The passengers were trying to escape while the seawater was rising in the cabin.
3. Accident victims often report imagining a worst version of the accident they survived. This may trigger panics: 'I could smell the petrol and imagined the car catching fire.'
4. Chronic illness patients, depressed medical patients or those with various medical phobias can flashforward to anticipated illness, disability or death, or an imaginary scene of their family alone. For example, diabetic patients may imagine themselves with an amputated leg.
5. In a sexual health clinic, patients may request repeated tests for human immunodeficiency virus after some sexual misadventure. Such a patient may report a flashback to the misadventure. ('The condom broke with that girl in South Africa'). There may be a flashforward to themselves dying of acquired immunodeficiency disease as they imagine it.

A judgement is required about the probability of the expected disaster. A patient with chronic illnes reported a flashforward of being trapped at home, unable to leave the house. This was unlikely, but a pessimist could not exclude it. In this case, the patient said that this situation would damage his marriage. When he discussed this with his wife, she told him his fear was unjustified. If the future event is a real thing and not imaginary, distress may not reduce beyond the reasonable level or may reverse in the future. Eye movement treatment is not contraindicated by the possibility that the effect may reverse at a later stage. Flashforwards are often associated with panics. Flashforwards are a special case of a symbolic or imaginary target.

7.5 SYMBOLIC, IMAGINARY OR RECONSTRUCTED

Distress images can be symbolic or in some other sense not real. The patient should be able to report that the image is not real. Eye movement desensitization does not require the flashback to be veridical. A patient may report distressing flashbacks of abuse at the age of four. We know accurate memories cannot be retrieved from that age, and so these are probably later reconstructions. This does not mean the patient was not abused at that age or that the flashback should not be treated. Some other examples are:

1. Patients will imagine their families in an accident, assault or trauma event similar to their own.
2. A parent may report imagining images of a child's assault or rape (post-traumatic stress disorder by proxy).
3. Due to hospital error, a man had the curious misfortune of reading the report of his late wife's autopsy. He then suffered from nightmares of being present at his wife's autopsy.
4. A patient survived a serious accident at work. He required eye movement treatment for the accident and painful episodes in treatment. He focused on a flashback of intense pain, followed suddenly by anaesthesia and a floating

feeling. He could look down on his crisis. This image had a high distress score. After some treatment, he decided to retain the less distressing image on the reasonable grounds that an 'out of body' experience should be remembered.

7.6 REPROCESSING

This is the reprocessing part of the full title 'eye movement desensitization and reprocessing'. The term is used here to describe the report of cognitive and emotional change, but without a distress reduction. There is an implication that distress reduction will occur later because of the reprocessing. As a guide, if four sets of eye movements go by without change, then consider if this is not reprocessing, and the flashback is not desensitizing, or is blocked. However, an apparently unchanged distress score may depend on how narrowly the flashback is defined.

A patient in desensitization of a house fire became blocked and required decomposition into different sensory modalities, as described in the next chapter. These images included the noise, the smell and the taste of the smoke. The taste sensation started high and then stabilized at a score of six. After this showed no change over ten sets, the patient was questioned more closely and reported 'I could feel the taste of the smoke in my mouth'. When asked for a strength of feel-of-taste score, six was reported, which was then zeroed. When this roadblock was cleared the other sensory targets also reduced.

7.7 LOW-SCORING FLASHBACKS

In treatment, a flashback may not desensitize below a certain score. As a guide, this means distress scores below four and they are usually about one or two. These must not be neglected, but they are of several types. First, note that such flashbacks might not yet be low-scoring. During assessment or treatment, the patient may report an apparent low score. However, relabelling with a different emotion may increase distress. Always focus on the highest score. Two examples are:

1. A patient being treated for panics may report a low anxiety score. However, when asked how embarrassing the panic was, it will be rated higher.
2. A rape victim may report a low anxiety score. If then asked to measure disgust, self-blame or humiliation, she or he may report a high score.

After these possibilities are checked, genuine low flashbacks remain an issue. The simplest case is a low-scoring flashback that appears in a series of high-scoring targets. This may not need individual treatment. This is because treating the high-scoring flashbacks may desensitize related lower-scoring ones. A reassessment after the high flashbacks are treated will demonstrate this.

A low score may not mean that a flashback is defused. In Chapter 9, it is asserted that eye movement therapy unloads the overloaded working memory. Any continuing restriction of working memory capacity may maintain the problem. Unless there is a good reason, all eye movement targets must be zeroed. An analogy is that a patient must always finish a course of antibiotics even if the symptoms of the infection have gone away, because some bacteria may still be alive at that point. The patient's mental hygiene is optimized by killing all flashbacks.

I suspect, from clinical experience, that low-scoring flashbacks can cause depression and sexual dysfunction. One woman's ten-year sexual dysfunction was cured with a 20-minute session on low-scoring intrusive memories of a life event with no apparent sexual implications. This event had occurred ten years earlier.

There may be a good reason why an eye movement sequence results in a stable low score. The flashback may have reached the level that makes sense in the patient's circumstances. I will call this the 'reasonable' level. Other similar expressions are the ecological level or natural level for that flashback. Often this is signalled by an inability to change cognition. The cognitions will have a rational relation to the situation, rather than a pessimistic one and cannot change any more. A real-world constraint on the situation has been reached. Such a flashback will not shift with further treatment. A few more sets on the target will test this, after suitable discussion. Some other action may then be indicated. For example, an assault patient stopped her treatment at low scores. We agreed that she had to decide if she should report the incident. She returned after reporting to the police and did not need any more treatment.

Similarly, a patient may rate fear of surgery at ten, and still have to face that surgery. In this situation, the flashforward of surgery will not reduce it below a fear score of three or four. One patient had severe, continuing and undiagnosed medical problems. He presented with distressing flashbacks of awareness during surgery. He had experienced great pain during surgery before managing to communicate with the anaesthetist. Eye movement desensitization included flashbacks of the surgical procedure. Treatment reduced the flashbacks to low scores, but no further. Since the medical situation was deteriorating, still unexplained, and required further investigation, this was the reasonable level. However, the patient then coped with a recent emergency admission without panicking and was able to admit to further symptoms.

One important version of this is bereavement flashbacks. Bad life events commonly involve a death. This may be witnessing the death of a family member, somebody who was killed in an accident or discovered after suicide. It may be that the patient wishes to retain some of this memory, but at some level less distressing than presented. With such a flashback, the patient can decide when treatment stops. Eye movement desensitization is sufficiently precise that this option exists. This option is explained in the briefing, or in the treatment if the issue appears. Sometimes other good memories of the deceased may come forward as the bad retreat.

7.8 BODY IMAGE

Another kind of image is the patient's body image with a real or imagined disfigurement. Eye movements can desensitize body image distress [85]. We should distinguish between body image distress and the body image distortion found in eating disorders. This is probably a different thing. The patient focuses on her body image in some way that arouses anxiety, which is then treated like a flashback: 'Please imagine being at home and looking at your body naked in the mirror.' I say 'her' specifically because men rarely report this. Examples might be scars or obesity seen in a mirror, or immediately after surgery, or with people looking at it. A case series shows that body dysmorphic syndrome can be treated in this way [86]. Body image checks may be required with female sexual assault victims. The patient is asked either as above, or a more explicitly sexual version. For example: 'Does the image of your genitals inspire disgust or fear?' A similar request may be: 'Please imagine being intimate with your husband.'

The strange-face-in-the-mirror illusion

Patients with body image issues should be warned not to examine themselves in the mirror for too long. After about ten minutes, the looker will perceive an illusion in which the face becomes deformed or distorted. The looker may perceive their face as having become distorted into that of another person or an animal [87]. This cannot be helpful to those concerned about their appearance.

7.9 PHOBIAS

Simple phobias can present with visual eliciting stimuli. This could be a flashback, such as a squashed spider or something that regularly occurs, such as finding a spider in the bath. Assessment should pursue the first, worst and most recent exposures to the eliciting stimulus. Phobias appear to be simple, but may not be. A patient with a swimming phobia reported flashforwards of each sensory experience of swimming: the noise, the smell of the sea, the feel of the water on her face and losing touch with the beach from under her feet.

7.10 INCOMPLETE FLASHBACKS

Patients may report only one or two of the three parts of the target: image, bad thought or emotion and physical feelings. This does not matter if we conflate cognitions, emotions and feelings into the same category. There may be just a report of unlabelled distress or physical sensation. A woman initially reported disgust as both cognition and physical sensation, but no specific image of her sexual abuse history. Another sexual abuse case focused on the anxiety that it would happen again, with a strong physical nausea. There may be a bad thought by itself: 'I am scared the panic will never go away.' The author has focused a patient on 'that guilty feeling' with success. Eye movements can be focused on such reports. A better report may appear in a few sets.

7.11 BE DIRECTIVE SOMETIMES

The therapist can be directive about flashbacks. A summary target can be suggested to test for distress. Patients can be asked to think of the accident or assault as a whole. Road traffic accident victims can be asked to imagine themselves driving or being in whatever position they were travelling in when the accident happened. Victims of assaults can be asked to imagine the face of the assailant, abuser or rapist. As described above, sexual assault victims can be directed to imagine their lower body image, or sexual relations.

Social phobia is treatable with eye movement desensitization. All patients with assault or rape reports, or between about 13 and 30 years of age, should be checked for it. Ask the patient to imagine these scenes:

1. *Imagine you are at a meeting or in a class. You have to stand up and talk or present a lecture. Everybody is looking at you and you think they think you are rubbish in some way. How scary is that?*
2. *You go to a party where you do not know anybody. You go in the room and everybody stares at you.*
3. *Imagine you are in a market on Saturday morning, when it is crowded.*

7.12 PRIMARY AND SECONDARY EYE MOVEMENT TARGETS

It is helpful to divide clinical problems that can be solved with eye movement desensitization into primary and secondary. Primary indications are supported by the trials, putting aside for now any issues about such trials. There are also secondary indications, such as food and drug cravings, bad reactions to cancer chemotherapy, phantom sensations and pain, and tinnitus. All the issues above this section are primary. All the issues below are secondary.

In general, secondary indications do not have support from trials, with the exception of the phantom pain study summarized below. Eye movement desensitization should start with primary targets and proceed to secondary targets. Eye movement desensitization is helpful for a secondary indication if it follows on from the primary problems. For example, it may be possible to decrease phantom pain if it follows on from flashbacks of a traumatic amputation in an accident, but not to an amputation under general anaesthetic for medical reasons. Therefore, all primary images must be fixed before secondary images are attempted.

Some secondary targets are of theoretical interest because they demonstrate that eye movement desensitization is based on something more than normal narrative or rhetorical psychotherapeutic models or explanations.

7.13 SEXUAL HEALTH

Experience in a sexual health clinic shows that eye movement desensitization helps sexual dysfunction caused by anxiety or another psychological problems. It is possible that dysfunction can be caused by flashbacks of sexual misadventure in the wider sense than obvious assaults. For example, the first attempt at sexual intercourse may have been consensual but went wrong. This may be associated with embarrassment or shame. There may be a semantic memory of parental advice that sexual intimacy is best avoided for some reason. The flashbacks reported may not be obviously sexual but may still cause sexual problems. For men, psychogenic erectile dysfunction can be treatable with eye movement desensitization. Men can be focused on their performance anxiety, both past and anticipated. One man's premature ejaculation decreased with eye movements focused on his embarrassing previous misadventures.

In women, this kind of sexual dysfunction may go a step further to vulvodynia or dyspareunia. Vulvodynia is chronic vulval discomfort. The patient complains of burning and soreness, but not itching. Dyspareunia is pain during or after sexual intercourse. Women with pain during intercourse may report flashbacks back to vaginal trauma events. This does not have to be obvious, such as a rape or difficult birth. It could be a history of sexual infection or cancer at a relevant site. Such women are not necessarily depressed, anxious or with inexperienced men. It may be that only their sexual functioning is affected. The author's experience is that eye movement desensitization may help with this. This is not a claim that such issues are always psychological rather than medical. Such patients should first be assessed by a relevant clinic for any physical basis to the problem. Detecting physical pathology does not contraindicate eye movement therapy, but may limit the effect.

7.14 GAMBLING

There is some evidence that addictive behaviours can be treated with eye movements. Drug use is considered below (Section 7.21). Another possibility is gambling behaviour. There is a trial of eye movement desensitization with chronic gamblers [88]. However, the flashbacks treated are not described in the report, though apparently they were conventional flashbacks. The gambling was reduced. It may be possible to treat the gambling behaviour itself and the related cognitions. For example, a patient was asked to imagine the casino he attended and score his loss of control feelings.

7.15 CHRONIC PAIN

Eye movement desensitization is helpful for chronic pain patients. However, we need to be clear what we are aiming at. In a pain clinic, eye movement desensitization is initially indicated because many patients have acquired the pain from a bad life event, such as an accident. Writing the bad life events list leads on to images of painful treatment, bad pain episodes and medical misadventure, and to flashforwards of future surgery, disability or death. Medical and social anxieties are also common: 'Nobody can see I am in terrible pain.' All this can be analysed as distressing imagery. These patients will also report the usual other suspects, such as domestic abuse and bereavement. All chronic pain patients should be assessed and treated for such issues, before any approach is made to possible treatment of the pain. Doing this is often enough to move the patient on. Can the pain itself be an eye movement target? Protocols have been written for pain eye movement treatment which assume so [89,90].

The report of pain may move up or down with treatment of related flashbacks. The patient may report an increase in the pain at the site of injury: 'I can feel the pain in my legs, where I was trapped in the car crash.' This can be considered as a pain flashback, which can be assessed and treated in the same way as any specific sensory flashback. It may not go to zero if there are other reasons for pain at that site. Note that pain has two halves: intensity (how much pain) and effect (how badly the pain upsets the patient). If eye movement desensitization does not reduce the whole pain, the effect component should be assessed. For example, the pain may cause nausea, which may reduce with eye movements.

7.16 PHANTOM LIMB SENSATION OR PAIN

It would appear that eye movement therapy can reduce phantom sensation and pain after amputation. This was first reported at the case series level [91,92]. With phantom pain, the ordinary trauma flashbacks must be fixed first. For example, if the patient lost a limb in an accident, assess and deal with flashbacks of the accident first. The phantom sensation or pain is assessed and treated as any other target. Consider it as a pain flashback. Determine what words the patient uses to describe this and find the pain score for those labels. If the patient can do anything to increase the pain, ask him to do it during eye movement desensitization. For example, phantom finger pain may be increased by moving the remaining fingers of that hand. The phantom sensation or pain may decompose into separate targets. A leg may be reported in two positions, pain may progress to other sensations, or pain from a phantom leg ulcer may be reported. Caution the patient that there may be some return of the pain. If this happens, more eye movement desensitization can be tried but all the pain may not go away. There may be other reasons for pain in that site. Continuing medical problems will limit the result.

I hypothesize, from clinical experience, that eye movement desensitization will affect phantom sensation or pain only when it is secondary to flashbacks to the trauma event that damaged the limb. This might be an accident or previous pain or disability in the limb. A phantom sensation resulting from non-traumatic amputation, perhaps under general anaesthetic after a diagnosis of cancer, may not be affected by eye movements. There is a randomized controlled trial reported from Iran [93]. Sixty amputation patients with phantom pain were divided into 2 groups of 30. Both experimental and control groups received treatment as normal, such as medication, physiotherapy, mirror therapy, and psychotherapy. The experimental group took 12 eye movement sessions over 1 month. Treatment targets are listed as the injury memory, amputation operation, post-amputation difficulties and then pain sensations. The experimental group improved. Of 30, 14 lost all pain, 12 most pain and 4 had a small response. This was maintained at a 24-month follow-up. Pain scores and distress scores decreased from around seven to two. Only one of the control group showed slight improvement and average scores got slightly worse. This is an impressive result. Note relevant trauma memories are treated as well as the pain. Perhaps this indicates that phantom pain treatment should be promoted to be a primary target. However, I will leave it on the secondary list, to ensure primary flashbacks are treated first.

7.17 TINNITUS

We should note tinnitus here. This is phantom sounds in one or both ears. It may change when primary targets are treated. When primary targets are cleared, assess, score and treat each ear separately. Ask the patient to listen to the sound as the focus. This does not always work, but is worth trying. I cannot say if it helps tinnitus without primary flashbacks.

7.18 OTHER ILLNESS SYMPTOMS

Eye movement desensitization can be used for symptoms caused by the illness or disorder itself after the primary flashbacks to causes of the disorder are treated. Examples are:
1. Receiving a difficult or life-changing diagnosis.
2. Painful treatment such as dressing changes on open wounds.
3. Worst symptom episodes, or most painful.
4. Hospitalization, either medical or psychiatric.

5. Depression episodes.
6. Suicide attempts.
7. Self-harm, such as cutting arms.

Victims of bad life events may report distressing imagery from self-harm or suicide attempts. Treatment of these attempts is secondary treatment of the life event memories that inspired the self-harm in the first place. A patient with a history of arm cutting can describe and score the tension feelings preceding the cutting episodes. If they have scars, ask them to look at the scars.

Self-harming is a complex issue and perhaps it does not reduce to advice to do eye movement therapy on flashbacks of cutting one's arms. There is no trial that shows benefit and this advice is based on my clinical experience. I do not understand the motivation for doing this to oneself. Patients will describe a need to reduce tension, but I cannot empathize with the decision that the tension is worse than the pain or the need to wear long sleeves for the rest of one's life.

It is here that one of the pragmatic virtues of eye movement therapy is helpful. The therapist does not need to understand or empathize. Empathy, like insight, is neither compulsory nor essential. Eye movement desensitization directed at self-harm images, in the context of eye movement treatment of the primary abuse or anxiety, is helpful.

Depression episodes may show up as distressing images. The patient can be asked 'Where do you remember being most depressed?' This can be the distress image that is measured and treated. Because depression is the illness that leads to bad life decisions, an associated emotion may be embarrassment. ('I am embarrassed at being depressed in front of people and doing those dumb things.') One patient answered 'sitting in the kitchen' and this discussion resulted in the decision to repaint the kitchen.

Patients with a chronic illness may have flashbacks to the worst episodes of the illness symptoms. This might be an episode of severe pain, a risk to their life or of receiving the diagnosis. There may not be any other bad life events, just the illness. Another possibility is that eye movement therapy could help with a cancer patient's reactions to cancer drugs. I have desensitized a cancer patient to the nausea triggered by domestic cleaning fluids, which were a reminder of chemotherapy.

7.19 DOMESTIC TRIGGERS

It is possibe to help with a class of distress triggers that sometimes appears in a series of images usually concerning illness. The patient will report difficulties with a family member. A parent, made vulnerable by illness or pain, can report difficulties with an adolescent child. An image can be requested of a typical confrontation incident, or the most recent or worst, and a 'tense feeling' score requested. This can usually be decreased to a safer level. Explain that this will not change the dissident teenager, but cooling the parental reactions makes it easier to deal with situations. Cooler parental reactions may lead to cooler offspring reactions. Discuss the antecedents and consequences of such behaviour. However, this should not be mistaken for family therapy. A similar situation is the patient after a marital break-up receiving verbal abuse or other misbehaviour from the almost ex-spouse over financial or child custody issues: 'Can you hear his voice on the phone in your mind's ear?' Work-stress triggers, such as a difficult boss, can be similar.

7.20 MORALLY LOADED FLASHBACKS

Some flashbacks will have implications for the patient that involve the problem of good, bad or personal responsibility. I use the term 'morally loaded' to describe this problem. Three examples are:

1. A soldier who killed somebody by mistake, perhaps a legitimate enemy, but perhaps a civilian or a child.
2. A patient who self-destructs a marriage as a response to a difficult bereavement.
3. A patient who, having been a victim of wartime atrocities, is then forced to inflict similar acts or be killed.

Alternatively, the patient may have been the victim and suffered some irreconcilable loss. Such morally loaded targets may not desensitize with eye movement therapy at first. If at a high distress score, possible solutions are described in Chapter 8, but they only work up to certain limits. Such memories may reduce to low-level flashbacks at the reasonable level. Beyond this, the patient's moral jeopardy or injury is too great and progress will stop. The only solution at this point is not to treat this flashback.

Subsequently, the situation will resolve into three possible alternatives. First, treatment can continue on the other flashbacks in the patient's series. If there is a close association between flashbacks, then treating related flashbacks will indirectly desensitize the difficult flashback. This is the neural network effect. In one such case, a patient reported a difficult flashback that had a distress score of 10 and could not proceed. After the associated flashbacks were reduced, this was then rated at five. The patient was then able to consent to a successful treatment on this flashback. Second, is that the limits of eye movement therapy have been reached and another method should be tried. This might be an opportunity to review and practise skills in the more reflective rhetorical methods. However, there is the risk of reaching the third alternative, which is that the limits of all therapy methods have been reached. There is a point at which the patient's moral dilemmas and injuries are their own business and this is best acknowledged.

7.21 DRUG CRAVINGS

This is cravings for recreational or psychoactive drugs, cigarettes or alcohol. Again, all primary flashbacks should be fixed first. Such patients often begin by self-medicating flashbacks of childhood abuse or other misadventures. Eye movement treatment may help reduce a drug craving, but that is only one part of giving up drugs. Reducing cravings helps only those people who have committed not to use again. Assess the drug craving target in some way. Some examples are as follows:

1. A cigarette craving may be reported after a domestic conflict.
2. An alcohol craving may be experienced when the patient walks by a pub and smells the pub smell, or when alone at home and depressed. One patient described a return of alcohol cravings when encountering somebody withdrawing from heroin.
3. Someone who has previously used street drugs may get a craving when they encounter a preparation and injection kit, or when they walk past the house of their supplier.
4. The patient may be focused on a flashforward of some imaginary utopia where no drugs of choice are available. I have asked such patients to imagine all the alcohol and cigarette shops have gone out of business and no supplies are obtainable.

Patients will use labels such as 'jittery' or 'edgy' to describe the craving. Reported cognitions may concern loss of control or panics. This is scored and used as the eye movement target. In one case, such craving-cued panics were being self-medicated with alcohol. This required each to be treated alternately, rather than treating the panics first as advised above. In my experience, such treatment does result in a reduction of use, but it needs to be reassessed and repeated several times. Some drug users seem unable to describe their problem in such terms. This may be because they have never reduced their intake to that point at which a craving occurs.

A note of caution is required here. I attempted eye movement therapy on a craving target with a long-time heroin addict, then on a methadone prescription. This patient had completed treatment for his abuse. He then reported flashbacks of episodes of attempting to detox himself at home, with uncomfortable and embarrassing physical reactions. In the session, he experienced all the physical reactions of withdrawal again. He was maintained on the target through a difficult session until some decrease was observed. He did not attend his next appointment and dropped out of treatment. I advise caution in such cases.

A trial of alcoholic patients in which eye movement therapy was directed at the craving (addiction memory) compared to normal inpatient treatment showed a superior reduction of cravings, with some maintenance, after a month [94]. However, as the report acknowledges, earlier life events were not treated. All life history flashbacks should be treated first. Eye movement desensitization can be either distress memory focused or addiction trigger focused. The advice given in this book is that distress memories are primary and are treated first. Addiction memories and craving triggers are secondary. However, it may not be possible to separate primary from secondary in a particular case. Perhaps the craving triggers panics. For review and advice, see Markus et al. [95].

7.22 FOOD CRAVINGS

It is possible food cravings can be treated in a similar way when dietary challenges or comfort eating are reported. Patients are focused on trigger situations, such as being at home depressed and desiring chocolate or seeing doughnuts in a supermarket, and asked to imagine they are forbidden to eat or buy. For one diabetic patient, this procedure stopped chocolate consumption and resulted in immediate improvements in physical health.

7.23 NIGHTMARES AND SLEEP PARALYSIS

Distressing imagery and symptoms can be experienced in the dark as well as in the light. Patients may report bad dreams, nightmares or waking with panics. These should be assessed and treated. Such dreams may clearly relate to a bad life event, or may not. Dreams do not need to be interpreted as a narrative. A distressing dream image of being chased by an unidentified assailant should be treated, without requiring identification of the abusive father. Discussing sleep disturbances may lead to the important issue of sleep paralysis. In Chapter 10, on biological explanations, the three wake and sleep stages are considered. We exist in three states:

1. With our bodies and brains awake.
2. In rapid eye movement sleep, with our bodies asleep and our brains dreaming.
3. In non-rapid eye movement sleep, with our bodies asleep and our brains less active.

For some people, on occasion, this goes wrong and the body remains asleep, while the brain gets stuck in one of the three states. This results in a feeling of being paralysed, with a weight on the chest, other body sensations, including sexual, and the opinion that something or somebody dangerous is in the room. This is the origin of the myth that people are visited at night by a demon, vampire, alien or angel [96]. Sleep paralysis is often the missing piece in the stranger or inexplicable presentations. It should be explained to the patient, since understanding is half the cure. This should also discourage any possible literary or religious inspiration.

Sleep paralysis should be distinguished from bad dreams, nightmares, night panics or real night-time events or sexual assaults. Another link may be with medical symptoms. Symptoms involving chest pain or breathing difficulties may indicate sleep paralysis. A review of 42 research reports on sleep paralysis summarizes as follows [97]. There is no difference by sex or age. Lifetime prevalence is between 6% and 9% in normal populations. This rises to 50% or 60% in pathological populations. Prevalence of sleep paralysis increases with panics, post-traumatic stress disorder, bad life events, other sleep disorders, and bad sleep habits such as too much or too little sleep. Sleep paralysis increases with bad physical health measured in general, but no specific illness except chronic pain.

I estimate about half of my patients report this. For our purposes, nightmares and sleep issues indicate that enquiry should be made for the symptoms above. A sleep paralysis episode will be reported as a flashback and should be assessed as an eye movement desensitization target. Experience shows that sleep paralysis goes away as the series of flashbacks is treated. After this, evaluate the experience of lying awake paralysed as an image and treat that. Eye movement desensitization is not a cure for sleep paralysis in that there is a trial to justify this, but my experience is that it does go away. Note that one patient reported an increase in sleep paralysis during treatment, but it was discovered that the improvement had led to a reduction in sleep medication, revealing the issue. I cannot say if this would help sleep paralysis without a history of trauma.

7.24 PSYCHOTIC SYMPTOMS

I began treating such patients when a patient with bipolar psychosis requested treatment for sexual assault memories. This patient was stable on medication, and was a clinical professional and thus aware of the issues. The treatment was successful and included flashbacks to the worst bipolar illness episodes. Another patient with schizophrenia was treated successfully for sexual and physical assault issues. I then directed eye movement therapy at the distressing memories of auditory hallucinations and then at the hallucinations themselves. There was a reduction in fear and loudness but not frequency. Once the primary trauma memories are reduced, can eye movement desensitization reduce psychotic symptoms as secondary targets?

Advice on treating psychotic patients can be found in Van den Berg et al. [98]. A large trial showed that both prolonged exposure and eye movement desensitization reduced psychological trauma symptoms in chronic psychotics [99]. There was no change in auditory hallucinations or paranoid thoughts. I cautiously postulate eye movement desensitization is safe to use with psychotic patients. However, the patient must be stable, on medication and be able to consent.

8. DEALING WITH PROBLEMS

8.1 STALLED FLASHBACKS

A flashback that does not change over four sets of eye movements is blocked or stalled. Similar problem flashbacks change slowly or show an increase in distress. For comparison at this stage, the four alternative outcomes are:

1. The expected decrease in symptoms (desensitization).
2. Reporting cognitive or emotional change without change of distress level or desensitization (reprocessing).
3. The recollection of previously unreported information, sometimes with distress and physical sensation.
4. No change of any type (stalled).

In this chapter, solutions for such problems are identified and discussed separately. In practice, they will overlap and combine together. Two examples are:

1. A patient reported flashbacks of watching violence between their parents as a child, became panicky with strong physical symptoms, and said, 'It will never go away'.
2. A road traffic accident victim completed eye movement desensitization to flashbacks of the accident in two sessions. It then became apparent he was still panicking while driving. Further treatment of this became blocked and the patient became distressed. He was asked: 'Can you imagine the accident happening again?' The patient became more distressed and replied 'yes'. Treatment on this flashforward again became blocked. The patient then reported a further sound flashforward to the sound of the crash. Eye movements then worked.

Two remedies for such problems are found in the training courses and other books. These are the safe-place procedure and teaching other distress control methods. The safe-place procedure is to identify a personal safe image from the patient's experience before eye movement desensitization. A patient who becomes distressed is asked to retreat mentally to this personal safe image.

I once had an instant version of the safe place. On the wall of my consulting room, I had a poster of dolphins jumping through the waves. I would tell distressed patients to imagine they were a dolphin. This worked quite well, but became redundant. Using the safe-place method does not actually treat the source of the problem. It is like a surgeon who encounters a bleed during an operation and responds by sewing the patient up and pronouncing the patient safe. It is made redundant by the advice below.

Other distress control methods, such as relaxation, could be taught. The reason not to do this is the use of alternative methods before eye movement desensitization vitiates any advantage from this innovation. Because eye movement desensitization is an improvement on previous methods, then using other methods before necessity is a waste of clinical time. I would also argue that such methods are a retreat from eye movement desensitization therapy. It is not a solution to problems that arise during the procedure.

My advice here is mostly based on the idea that post-traumatic stress disorder, anxiety and chronic distress are proximally caused by overloaded working memory and this happens in a neural network (see Chapters 9 and 10). If there is a problem, it is usually caused by working memory restricted capacity, which becomes overloaded and blocked. The consequence is distress and the treatment stalls. An analogy is threading a needle. If the thread will not go into the eye of the needle, then we use either a smaller thread or a bigger needle. One remedy is to reduce the size of the eye movement desensitization target until it fits into the patient's memory capacity. Another is to treat easier flashbacks, giving more working memory bandwidth for the difficult flashbacks. Consider the following solutions.

8.2 REASSESS

The first thing to do with a stalled flashback is to reassess it. The simplest solution is that the flashback has changed and the patient has not told you for some reason. There may be another higher-scoring flashback that should take priority. Reassess this flashback, then proceed. Sometimes, treatment initially fails with several flashbacks, and a series has to be tried before one yields. A rape victim made slow progress on the usual flashback such a patient reports. After questioning her in more detail about her symptoms, she reported tension in her shoulders, caused by the physical feeling flashback of the rapist holding her down by the shoulders. Eye movement desensitization applied here worked and the earlier targets then made progress. Sometimes, the patient is just a bad reporter and needs careful questioning after each set.

8.3 DECOMPOSE THE FLASHBACK

The take-home advice of this chapter is that most problems in eye movement desensitization can be solved by breaking the target down into smaller chunks. Each then becomes one flashback or target. This new flashback might seem trivial compared with the whole trauma narrative, but is required to bootstrap the process. The right flashback is the one that changes with eye movements. There are six ways to achieve this:

1. Decompose a semantic memory into episodes. A patient who has been regularly assaulted in some way for years will not remember every episode. Such a patient is asked to focus a big general memory of the regular assault, but gets stuck at a distress score of 7 (S= 7). Enquire if one episode stands out as worse, perhaps the first or last.

2. Divide the timeline of an episode up, so that the stalled target is separated out into a sequence of two, three or more flashbacks. A better focus is found on the sequence of events. We can call this the horizontal method, to compare with the vertical.

3. The third or vertical method separates a flashback into the different sensory modalities. If we assume the flashback was visual and the treatment stops, try asking about sound or smell flashbacks. For example, a traffic accident may be divided into the sound, the physical sensation or pain from the moment of impact, or the smell of petrol. Sensory-specific images can be episodic or semantic. Here are some examples of sensory-specific flashbacks:

(3.1.) A soldier discovered a booby-trap bomb in a car that his patrol were investigating. They ran away and the bomb exploded behind them. The pressure wave picked him up and threw him on the ground several yards away. In this case, the noise, the flash and the sensation of flying through the air were separate targets.

(3.2.) A patient may be focused on the sound flashbacks of the words used: 'I can hear my father shouting at me that it would make my mother worse unless I had an abortion.' This can be the patient's own voice: 'I can hear myself screaming at the nurses when they tried to control me in a manic episode.'

(3.3.) There may also be pain or sensation flashbacks experienced at the site of the injury or assault: 'I can feel pain on the side of my head where my father used to hit me.' Treating a rape may require separate focus on penetration pain and sensations.

(3.4.) Childhood sexual abuse victims commonly report that the abusing male adult ejaculated during the abuse, perhaps onto their face or into their mouth. In this case, the patient may have to be focused on the smell or taste of seminal fluid.

Distress triggers like these can be explicit. The good therapist will help their patients through these flashbacks as fast as possible, without getting distressed, angry or disgusted on behalf of the patient. The author finds it helpful on these occasions to imagine one is a brain surgeon removing a tumour.

4. The fourth method of flashback decomposition is to use a systematic desensitization hierarchy. Systematic desensitization requires the anxiety trigger to be decomposed into a series of progressively more distressing triggers. The first will score low on the distress scale and the rest rise up a ladder of progressively more distressing triggers. A spider phobia might be broken down into small passive spiders and progress up to large active ones. A stalled flashback could be decomposed into a similar ladder. This is the opposite of the advice to start with high-distress flashbacks and work down. However, sometimes such a gentle approach may be a good idea. For example, a patient with a history of sexual assault could not make any progress with a flashforward of intimacy with her good second husband. She showed high distress imagining this. I asked her to focus on this, considering that it indicated the

correct target. However, she made no progress. Progress began when her imagined encounter was broken down into stages of his arrival (low distress score), his approach to her (slightly higher distress), etc.

5. The fifth method of image decomposition is found in body image desensitization. A body image can be divided into the back and front views, or a scar, operation site or amputation stump. Treatment of a colostomy image can be divided into the stoma by itself and with the colostomy pouch.

6. The last method of image decomposition is found in body sensation desensitization. I will call this anatomical decomposition. For example, assault victims report physical sensations, or pain, from the assault. The report can be decomposed by asking the patient to focus on different parts of the body separately. This can be symmetrical. A patient may report being held down by the shoulders. This patient can be asked to focus the left shoulder sensation and then the right shoulder. A patient who had his face held required focus on the left and then right side of his face.

8.4 MOVE ON CREATIVELY

If no other solution works with a stalled flashback, then leave it alone and proceed in another direction. There are various ways of doing this. The first is simply to move to another flashback. If flashback number 1 cannot be treated, move onto flashback number 2. It may be that number 2 seems trivial compared with number 1, but that does not matter. It may be that a series of flashbacks, numbers 2 to 7, have to be cleared before number 1 can be moved. This advice is based on the premise that eye movements unload a blocked or overloaded working memory. Desensitizing number 2 (to number 7) will provide more space in working memory for number 1. In the threading the needle analogy, this is like using a needle with a bigger eye, because we do not have a smaller thread.

Sometimes potentially difficult material can be avoided altogether. A woman reported extensive child abuse from a family member. During treatment, she also reported the death of her first child from a common infection. This was distress scored at ten. This was noted, but not desensitized. At the last appointment, all abuse flashbacks had been reduced to zero. The child's death had reduced to a distress score of 3 with no direct work. She reported this as the correct level. This is the working memory effect. As working memory capacity is increased, the patient is enabled to self-desensitize distress memories. The resource we are installing is working memory space.

8.5 UNCLOSED SESSION

An unclosed session means that flashbacks that have opened up have not been worked through and closed down. This may be caused by the discovery of difficult flashbacks late in the session when there is not the time to work through as advised above. This can be as much about timing as difficulty. The patient can be taken through a simple relaxation routine or otherwise calmed down in some way. The experienced eye movement therapist can reflect at this difficult time that other methods probably upset the patient more often.

This often looks worse than it is. If the treatment has liberated enough working memory bandwidth, the patient will continue to process bad memories outside the session. One patient recalled a painful flashback of his medical history. He became angry and left treatment. He would never enter the hospital again. A few years later, he approached the author to report he was having further medical treatment. He now approved of eye movement desensitization and was recommending it to his friends.

8.6 SEVERAL OTHER POSSIBILITIES

Several other practical possibilities should be kept in mind. Sometimes eye movement desensitization is too fast and a session should be stopped before the planned finish. The patient needs a break to catch up and consider the situation. This might be five minutes within the session or five years between appointments. It may be that eye movement therapy should be stopped and another method of 'eye movement' desensitization tried. These other methods of sensory stimulation are considered below. Maybe a mistake has been made and this patient should not be having eye movement desensitization. Always be aware of this possibility and be prepared to withdraw gracefully. Sometimes the patient is assessed on a bad day. Sometimes the initial assessment provides enough exposure to the problem that the patient no longer needs eye movement desensitization.

There can be other problems. For example, one patient did not like or cooperate with authority figures. Eye movement desensitization did not work and it is possible the author had been mistaken for an authority figure. Another refused further treatment when it caused a flare-up of pain in the injury caused by the accident.

Sometimes a stalled flashback just needs further information or action to resolve it. Here are some examples. A patient with a history of assault could not permit an examination to detect a suspected medical issue. After several sessions, the necessary medical exam was consented to and performed. No physical anomaly was found. Similarly, a patient may stop treatment to sort out an issue. One patient stopped treatment and asked me to obtain her medical file. When this was read and discussed, she decided she had finished treatment.

8.7 CHECK THE BAD THOUGHTS

Certain problems involve a cognitive or emotional label on a flashback. We recall from an earlier discussion that eye movement desensitization does not require a coherent negative automatic thought that causes an emotion, as required for cognitive therapy. Just reporting the raw emotion is enough.

Checking on the bad thoughts requires three things:

1. Has it changed? This might be either the cognition or the emotion.
2. Is the change good, bad or worse?
3. Is the change important or trivial?

The eye movement process may stop if the cognitive or emotional label fails to make sense with the image. The next label must be assessed. This may be a simple change from anxiety to disgust. Expect an increase in distress score with such a change. Once the change is determined, the patient can be refocused and moved on. For example, a road traffic accident victim's panic was triggered by a flashforward of a future accident. This did not change very fast until the following self-statement was reported: 'I don't want this to happen again.' Then progress became faster.

The patient may not report a coherent cognition or emotion. If other evidence of improvement is seen, such as convincing distress reduction, do not insist on it. Proceed, and cognitive change may then be reported. Patients may just need a short period of self-reflection between sets, rather than a formal label defined. It is necessary to be sensitive to the various labels that people use for their distress. Three to be careful with are embarrassment, humiliation and shame. Embarrassment is commonly associated with distress symptoms, notably panic attacks. Humiliation or shame appears when the patient believes, rightly or wrongly, that their performance in a difficult situation has not been adequate for their job description as a soldier, parent, big sister or whatever.

It is possible to miss the importance of a change of cognition. The therapist may assume a report is positive and miss the significance to the patient. A report may not initially be understood as negative. If in doubt, ask if this is a good thought or a bad thought. A change in the positive direction may throw up a negative cognition that causes a problem. Here are two examples.

1. A patient from a road traffic accident that happened with his wife in the car reported a flashback that included the wife screaming with fear (she was not injured). When this sound flashback was decreased, he became panicky, telling himself this meant the wife was being taken away and he would not see her again. When I understood this, I was able to persuade him that a disappearing flashback was a good thing and the eye movement desensitization worked again.

2. A patient did eye movement desensitization for an episode of acute and disabling pain, which proved to be the first sign of a serious illness. On this first occasion, friends and family came to his aid and called an ambulance. At a certain point, eye movement treatment had disappeared the helpers but not the pain memory. The bad thought then became 'I'm on my own' and anxiety increased. Eye movement was successful when maintained on the changed target.

Sometimes the personal, legal and moral implications cause the cognitions to change fast between each set. This process needs to be monitored carefully, often between each set. One example was a male patient who reported adolescent homosexual events as abuse, while admitting being uncertain about his own sexuality. As the treatment proceeded, he began to acknowledge that the encounter was less abusive than he had previously thought, because perhaps he was homosexual. Change will continue if the target is refocused between each set, but expect to reach the reasonable level.

One common problem is that the label may have a self-referential or catastrophizing quality. Here, the patient is commenting on the effect of the trauma rather than any other label. The bad thoughts have a pessimistic relation to the situation, rather than rational. If the patient is concerned about being rude about the therapist's efforts to help, this may be difficult to elicit. Some examples are:

1. 'I feel as if I am blocking it.'
2. 'I can't block it out.'
3. 'I am never going to get rid of this picture.'
4. 'I do not want to look at it; it is too scary/bad/sad.'
5. 'It is part of me after all this time.'
6. 'This is so bad, it will never change.'
7. 'I could remind myself of it if I wished.' (Read back from notes to test this.)
8. 'Nothing is going to work for me.'
9. 'I can't get past this.'
10. 'If I lose the flashback, I might go back to him.' (Said by an abused woman of her husband.)
11. 'I can't imagine this being painless.'
12. 'If I go out by myself, I will panic.' (This may indicate a flashforward to future panics.)

The solution here is to focus the patient on the flashback with the self-referential cognition as the new label. Ask for any physical sensation. The solution is not, at the risk of sounding unsympathetic, to sympathize with the patient or agree with the pessimism. Any logical discomfort caused by the self-referential nature of such bad thoughts is not a reason to stop eye movement desensitization. This apparent logical problem does not need a narrative solution. This is not the moment to agree the world is a bad place or to see the patient as a symbol of oppression. This problem must be distinguished from reasonable cognitions concerning a continuing difficult situation.

8.8 PANICS

Panics are important. If previous treatment results reverse in a later session, one explanation is that the patient is panicking between sessions. Panics may not show up in the assessment. One way of considering panics is that patients are re-traumatizing themselves, triggered by an internal cue rather than an external event. Assess the first , worst and most recent panic attack memories, treating them like flashbacks. The first and the worst will often be the same, but some patients will not remember their first attack. If the patient is having regular panic attacks, assess the most recent at each appointment, even though this may be different panic events.

It may be that morning, triggered by the prospect of discussing the matter. As the treatment of panic attacks proceeds, they may reduce to anxiety flare-ups without the physical symptoms that define panics. Reassessment of the flashback should change accordingly: 'Are you still having anxiety attacks?' Common themes in panics are:

1. Fear of death
2. Loss of control
3. Social embarrassment
4. Fear the panic attacks will not stop
5. Fear of future panics. Always test for flashforwards of future panics, perhaps in a particular place or situation: 'I am scared I will panic and die if I leave the house alone.'

Panics may wake the patient up at night or strike when they wake up. The physical sensation may be important and is commonly reported from under the sternum. It may be necessary to decompose the various triggers and sensations as described above. Some panics can be difficult and the panic triggers may require repeated treatment over several sessions. Frequent panics need frequent appointments to catch up with them.

Panics may be cued by another part of the problem, such as pain, sleep disturbances, sleep paralysis, drug cravings or distressing flashforwards. One patient with a bad history reported daily panic attacks and nightly bad dreams of his flashbacks. There were also panics at night caused by fear of the nightmares. This problem began to decrease only after some 15 sessions, which progressively decomposed the problem into 12 different targets. Those related to the difficult history were desensitized quickly, but those including panic attacks required repeated treatment. As in this case, some flashbacks will require repeated treatment, especially those with strong physical reactions. Sometimes, success is apparent only when a difficult, panicky or unstable flashback progressively requires less sets in subsequent sessions.

If the patient panics in the session, use the panic, especially the physical sensation, as the target. An accurate eye movement desensitization will reduce the panic set by set. If necessary, slow their hyperventilation between sets. Sometimes, a panic cue may work so fast it is difficult to target the panic symptoms themselves. Panic provocation is used in cognitive therapy to teach self-control and an eye movement provocation can be used in the same way. If this is not possible, consider it an unclosed session.

8.9 UNSTABLE FLASHBACKS

An unstable flashback has been desensitized in initial sessions, but retesting in subsequent sessions shows that it has activated again. There can be several reasons. The first is that the series of flashbacks is not yet fully reported or finished and the result will be stable when it is. If this does not happen, there are further reasons. The second is that the bad event is still happening for the patient. This takes us out of the territory of eye movement desensitization. A third possibility is that the patient is having panic attacks, as considered above.

The fourth possibility is that the patient has been avoiding treatment by not focusing on the trauma and moving on to the happy ending or another safe memory. This can be signalled by a large reduction in the distress score, usually of 4 or more points per set. It can be difficult to tell the difference between this and fast improvement. Both the test for this problem and the solution is to read back the flashback to refocus the patient on the danger signal. It may be necessary to repeat this each set if in doubt. Here are two examples.

1. A road accident victim showed a series of rises and falls of the distress score without reaching zero. Closer questioning revealed he was most anxious when he visualized himself sitting in the car, but his anxiety reduced if he was standing beside it. His distress level was decreasing by getting out of the car, not by eye movements. Treatment was successful only when he kept himself in the car.

2. A woman was trapped in a fire in a 400-year-old house with a heavy oak roof. A light modern ceiling had been installed inside the house. In the flashback, there was a crashing sound above and she was crushed to the floor. She thought it was the oak roof and that she would be dead. However, it was only the ceiling and she survived. Treatment failed over several sessions while the patient was allowed to follow the story through to the realization that it was only the ceiling. It worked only when she was repeatedly reminded, for each set, to focus on the crashing sound and the fear that the oak roof was coming down on her head.

8.10 DISSOCIATION IS NOT A PROBLEM

Dissociation is considered a problem in eye movement desensitization, but I am not clear why. I have never seen anything I recognize as, or need to call, dissociation in 29 years of practice of eye movement desensitization. Perhaps I do not permit my patients to dissociate. Consequently, I think that dissociation is not a problem. Am I right? If I am wrong why do I not see, or perhaps not recognize, dissociation? Perhaps I have been decomposing the flashback before dissociation happens.

If your author does not know what dissociation is, how can we find out? In Chapter 1, we noted that post-traumatic stress disorder came with two types of dissociation. Depersonalization is the feeling of being an observer, with time slowed down. Derealization is the feeling that the world is unreal, distant or distorted. I see no reason to treat such reports as a contraindication or additional pathology.

Other interpretations are possible. Depersonalization might just be the change of image perspective. If accompanied by distress, try one of the solutions given in this chapter. Other events called dissociative could be just memory failures. Such memory lapses may just be working memory issues, as discussed in Chapter 9. If a patient loses attention to the task, ask if they are still tuned in to what the therapist is saying. Possibly, the patient's attention will become so focused on internal physiological events that they lose attention to external events. If the patient says 'It felt like I was back there', reply 'That is why it is called a flashback.'

The argument I make here concerning dissociation is the same as I make for repression elsewhere. Dissociation can be just another word for repression. There is no need to privilege such events with a special name or action. A more careful comment about dissociation might be that the word is used for so many different events, it has no diagnostic utility, at least in our context. Any such event in treatment can be dealt with using the advice in this chapter. In our context, dissociation is another symptom of overloaded working memory.

In my opinion, much of the issue with dissociation is self-fulfilling prophecy. As best I understand this issue, there is concern that some disaster might ensue if the patient disassociates. One possible catastrophe that is anticipated might be dissociative identity disorder. This is the event formerly known as multiple personality disorder [100]. It can be found in the manual as the disruption of identity characterised by two or more distinct personality states, which may be described in some cultures as the experience of possession. I understand that some psychological therapists find a lot of this and some find none. I have seen something like it once, maybe, in 30 years, and it went away when I agreed with the patient that we would not do anything to compromise the patient's dignity. Those therapists who can see dissociative identity disorder, or who can see the patient's cognitions in different parts, or alters, which cannot communicate with each other without the therapist's help, can speak for themselves [101]. Critical reviews can be found in reference [102].

Beyond giving my opinion here, I will not attempt to summarize or discuss this issue further than necessary. The essential critique of dissociative identity disorder is that there is no logical necessity or even simple requirement to name any distress, symptom, behaviour, report or gap in narrative or memory, or a physiological or brain imaging anomaly as caused by another personality, alter or part. This is another failure of the narrative explanation. When the narrative of

Alice's problems runs out of narrative power, we discover Bob inside her and start a second narrative. Why should I want to tell Alice, suffering from panics, that there is another personality or alter inside her?

Perhaps in the pragmatic and utilitarian eye movement desensitization world I am trying to persuade the reader to enter, if you find another voice in the patient's head, then this is a sound flashback, perhaps to verbal abuse from an abuser. In the multiple personality world, this could be the beginning of another personality, perhaps with the allegation that the alter is based on the abuser. Perhaps Alice might want to label her internal sensations as Bob, not anxiety or tension, but it is not in Alice's interest to encourage this. We should also consider if Alice has a physical illness, sleep paralysis, panics, bipolar disorder or borderline personality disorder. Also, recall the advice about body image in Chapter 7, concerning the face in the mirror illusion. Perhaps Alice should be warned not to look for Bob or her other alters in the mirror. We should not multiply explanatory personalities, or parts thereof, beyond necessity. Perhaps such patients produce other personalities to avoid being abandoned by their therapist.

8.11 BORDERLINE PERSONALITY DISORDER MAY BE A PROBLEM

What is borderline personality disorder? Personality disorders are chronic behaviour and personal experiences that differ in distressing and damaging ways from those expected. There are 12 personality disorders noted in the manual [1]. The one that eye movement therapists are most likely to encounter is borderline personality disorder. These patients will attempt to avoid abandonment by other people, which may be either real or imagined. They may also have unstable personal relationships, impulsive behaviour and anger issues. There is a risk of self-harm or suicide.

Borderline personality disorder is commonly misunderstood such that the borderline being referred to is taken to be the border between normal and disorder, or illness. It is an old classification, originally founded in the opinion that neurotic patients could be cured by psychoanalysis. This is compared with psychotic patients, who did not benefit from psychoanalysis [103]. Some patients the psychoanalysts had issues with were not obviously psychotic, but still could not be helped by their methods. They were considered to be on the border between neurosis and psychosis. This problem can be solved by calling it emotionally unstable personality disorder.

The risk here is that a diagnosis by exclusion from the curable becomes a bin for the incurable. If one believes that psychoanalysis is effective for the neurotic, then failures who are not psychotic are called something else; that is, borderline personality disorder. It can be said that it borders other psychiatric illness, such as bipolar disorder. However, all psychiatric illness has high co-morbidity, so borderline personality disorder could border most things. Eye movement desensitization therapists are most likely to encounter such patients because they will report a history of trauma, usually, but not limited to, child abuse.

Should patients with borderline personality disorder receive eye movement desensitization? I have no doubt they commonly do. I have treated such cases, without disaster or harm. I suspect many such patients forget they have borderline personality disorder after good eye movement treatment and transform into normal trauma cases. My original opinion was that borderline personality disorder was a presentation of extensive child abuse or traumatic life history in patients who have tried to self-harm. Therefore they could receive eye movement desensitization.

This opinion is based on patients who present in medical clinics and report a past diagnosis of personality disorder when asked about previous illness. Often they do not seem to have received much help beyond the diagnosis or a place in the queue for dialectical behaviour therapy. The view from a personality disorder service might be different. There are cases where the patient has difficulty expressing distress and might self-harm to express this. There is the risk of a deceptive presentation. Consistent failure to improve in an eye movement treatment, despite all the advice in this chapter, might indicate personality disorder. As noted above, failure to improve was the original reason for this diagnosis.

There are no controlled trials at the moment of writing that support eye movement desensitization for borderline personality disorder. There is a case series that followed personality disorder patients who received eye movement desensitization, additional to their usual treatment [104]. Symptoms of post-traumatic stress, dissociation and insomnia reduced but no changes in auditory or verbal hallucinations or self-harm were found. For further advice, see this review by Mosquer et al. [105]. There are trials that support the use of certain cognitive therapy methods, not discussed further here. Remember the advice for such patients includes good liaison with other colleagues concerned with the case. There are limits to eye movement desensitization and such patients might find them.

8.12 NOT USING EYE MOVEMENTS

If eye movement therapy does not work, try a different method of 'eye movement desensitization' that does not depend on eye movements. This may seem initially confusing but that is because eye movements were the first method discovered that has this accelerated desensitization effect. Subsequently other similar methods have been identified. Depending on what we think eye movement desensitization is, then these other methods may work in a similar way. I will list the two I know here.

1. Sound. The sound can be bleeps, alternating between ears. There are devices available for this, which are battery-powered signal generators that feed into headphones. There are also audio files and apps available. There is evidence that eye movements are more effective than bleeps, but patients prefer bleeps [106].

2. Taps and vibrations. The same devices can feed a signal into tactile probes that vibrate. They are held in the hands, or between the hands and legs. Using your hands to tap

on the patient's hands works fine, but best not tried with an assault victim. During the Covid-19 lockdown, we have discovered that instructing the patient over video link to tap hands on legs also works.

8.13 WHEN NOTHING WORKS

It can happen that all solutions given here do not move the patient on. Perhaps the patient is distressed but unable to explain why. Possibly a problem has been reached that cannot be acknowledged for some reason. The eye movement therapy will be blocked until they do acknowledge it (which they might not). This can be difficult to deal with since you do not know what is happening. An unclosed session can result. These three examples were validated by later information:

1. A patient could not admit to being a victim of childhood abuse, despite successful treatment of combat memories.
2. A man could not admit to assaulting his wife.
3. A patient could not admit to possible symptoms of an illness that might prevent career plans.

Perhaps the patient is angry about some aspect of the trauma. The following script may help with this.

There are two sides to being angry. First, you may be morally right to be angry about what happened to you. It is not my job to make a judgement about that. However, if it had happened to me, I would probably feel the same way you do. Second, are you right to let the anger hurt you and block your recovery? It is my job to tell you that this should not happen and help you to stop that happening. I do not want you to think that I think you are wrong to be angry. One way of looking at it is that we will change your hot anger into cold anger.

Such problems may be insoluble in the eye movement desensitization world and require us to remember our previous skills.

8.14 RETREAT TO CONVENTIONAL METHODS

This comes last, since it should be considered last, when the procedural changes advised above have failed. Your author needs to confess here that for a long time, I understood the term 'cognitive interweave', to mean the retreat to cognitive methods described below. Chapter 10 of Shapiro's book corrected me. Cognitive interweave is a method of unblocking a treatment that has stalled. The therapist leads the discussion of the session to discover relevant cognitions, which are then encouraged by leading the patient through a set of eye movements. This is similar to the installation of positive cognitions method I attempted to discourage in Chapter 6. Since I have never needed to do this, then the procedural solutions above are sufficient.

In an eye movement desensitization session, the eye movement desensitization procedure has priority over other methods. However, some problems require a retreat to conventional methods. The best example is a blood or medical phobia, which has an anomalous physiological response requiring particular methods [107]. The patient may also produce a cognition that is sufficiently general that it stops eye movement desensitization. Cognitive or behavioural therapy is then required.

One example is the patient who believes that their other symptoms, perhaps of post-traumatic stress disorder or continued physical ill health, are the first signs of a mental breakdown. For example, a patient had a flashback to an incident of major blood loss. When he focused on this, he lost attention, began to faint and told himself this was the first sign of a worse problem. This was a blood phobia reaction, with further cognitive anxiety, which required treatment for a blood phobia, cognitive therapy and counselling, interweaved with further eye movement desensitization. This type of presentation can be obscure, such as a patient who panicked because the flashback included an episode of post-concussion amnesia. The associated bad thought was a fear of mental deterioration, made worse by current trauma memory problems. Ideally, such problems should be detected before eye movement treatment, but possibly the treatment causes a recollection of them.

The advice in this chapter is premised on the theory that we are unloading an overloaded working memory using artificial dreaming. This last section is the exception and considers what to do when we are obliged to operate inside a working memory that still might be overcrowded. The next two chapters look at working memory and artificial dreaming.

9. WORKING MEMORY

9.1 A USEFUL EXPLANATION

Even after 30 years of eye movement desensitization, many people are still troubled by it. This means it is either not used to the benefit of patients at all, or use is delayed while other methods are tried first. These methods presumably inspire less confusion. An explanation of eye movement desensitization might dispel this confusion.

Why should we use eye movement desensitization? Because it is an improvement or innovation on previous methods. If not an improvement, there would be no point in using it. How is it an improvement? My answer is that it is faster. It may have other virtues as well, but I will lead on faster. Faster means we can treat more patients per unit of health service money. This is good, because all health service budgets exist in the utilitarian frame of reference. We will not achieve this public good unless we use eye movement desensitization first, not last. If we use it last, after trying other methods that make us feel safer, then it is not an innovation, because there is no saving of clinic time. A convincing explanation is required [108]. When we move the patient's eyes from side to side, the decisions we make depend on what we imagine is happening in the patient's brain. This explanation of eye movement desensitization will control how we use it and what we think the possible risks and benefits are.

I propose we divide psychological therapy methods into rhetorical and procedural. 'Rhetoric' is a misused word. It can be derogatory, meaning a style of talking that is intended to impress but empty of substance. It can be this and one thinks of the statements of politicians. However, it has an older meaning, as the art of public speaking with the intention to impress, persuade or influence. This is a craft in itself, regardless of the merits of the case being presented. I am using the word to classify those methods that seek to improve the patients by verbal discussion, persuasion or teaching.

Most of what is called psychotherapy, and all of counselling, is rhetorical. All talking therapies are rhetorical. I wish to draw attention to the fact that talking, or teaching, is the tool a therapist uses to make a desired change. The words comprise the tool. This is in contrast to procedural methods, where the procedure is the tool used to make an improvement. I want to make this distinction because eye movement desensitization is a procedure.

We distinguish between rhetorical and procedural methods of psychological treatment to distinguish between explanations for rhetorical and procedural methods. I wish to dispute the idea that procedural therapies require the kind of rhetorical or narrative explanation that rhetorical therapies attract. Rhetorical methods aim to achieve insight because that insight will reduce distress and improve the patient's life.

Is insight necessary or sufficient? Insight is the subjective and narrative account of the reason for anxiety, distress or behaviour, found by introspection of the respondent's own thoughts. It is the knowledge the mind reports of the mind's reasons. However, insight is neither necessary nor sufficient to help the patient. Before eye movement desensitization, there was systematic desensitization, which is also a procedure. Systematic desensitization required relaxation and the imaginary climbing of a scale of anxiety triggers, monitored with anxiety scores. We could argue that these two methods are similar, except that eye movements are an improvement on relaxation and in eye movement desensitization, it is best to climb down the distress ladder, not up it. Systematic desensitization is effective. Trials in the 1960s showed it was superior to insight therapy [109].

Procedural methods can achieve insight, if all goes well, but do not require it as an active ingredient. Insight into meaningful connections is not, of logical necessity, evidence for causal connections. Connections between an event and the distress that a patient reports as meaningful may not be causal. Insight requires memory, which is less than perfect. Nobody is against insight, in the same way that nobody is against the environment or apple pie. There is no logical necessity to regard insight as a more powerful explanation, or lever for improvement, than images and tapping on sensory nerves in some way. Perhaps we can explain our problem by considering the effects of procedure or finding a way to detect a signal that acts as a clue.

The requirement for a procedural explanation can be confusing if one thinks that all behaviour, or action, is determined by explicit thoughts. There are many demonstrations that it does not have to be. For example, the distinction between declarative and procedural memory shows this. Procedural memory is the memory for procedures that are not declared, or put into words. The comparison between declarative and procedural memory and the distinction between rhetorical and procedural methods being advocated here is interesting, but probably just an analogy. There is no claim that procedural methods work on procedural memory, although this is an interesting speculation.

9.2 WHAT DO WE WANT FROM AN EXPLANATION?

One way into this problem is to ask what we want an explanation for. First, the explanation must accommodate the known facts. These are:

1. Most people recover from most bad life events without our help. Therefore, any explanation of recovery must not depend on the attention of the psychological therapist or the report of the patient. This is the paradox of post-traumatic stress disorder. Although the patient will express the problem as distressing memories, this does not explain

the cause of the problem, or at least, it is not the full explanation. The paradox is only superficial. It diminishes once we stop thinking in narrative terms.

2. In the general case, eye movement desensitization works if it is done correctly.

3. In the general case, eye movement desensitization gets easier as you continue.

4. When it works, cognitive change and relief of distress happens for free. By this I mean that improvement occurs in the patient's report of distress symptoms without direct verbal or rhetorical attention to them, other than that required to use the eye movement method.

5. Eye movements are not compulsory to eye movement desensitization. Other sensory stimulation methods are permitted. Any explanation must generalize beyond the visual system.

6. Eye movement desensitization may remedy problems other than those considered the province of a psychological therapist. Therefore, explanations other than those usually used are required.

Second, I want to set some conditions on the explanation:

7. Before embarking on this attempt at explanation, I want to lower the bar. No psychotherapy method has been explained satisfactorily, except those formulations and narratives that apply only to one person and not to the next patient in the waiting room.

8. To explain it fully, then we would have to understand 100% how the brain works. Since we are not going to achieve this soon, we must compromise. We should try to reach a level

of explanation that allows prediction and improvement.

9. The explanation should predict what to do next during treatment or how to solve problems.
10. The explanation should make sense to the patient.
11. We should not mistake a description of the problem for an explanation. Similarly, explanation does not consist of a list of possible or desirable components to achieve improvements, even if presented in boxes connected by arrows. Specifying the input and output of a black box is not explaining. We must try to reverse-engineer what is happening in the box, or at least speculate creatively.
12. A reductionist explanation is called for. Understanding a thing usually requires breaking the thing down to smaller pieces that we can understand.
13. Some separation of concepts may be a good thing.

These last three requirements are similar. It is my understanding that a scientific explanation requires breaking down an insoluble problem into smaller parts that become progressively more soluble. Perhaps smaller problems are easier to explain because we are familiar with them, by fact or analogy, or we can experiment with or observe something about them. Note that reducing a problem into smaller parts that we can do something with is like decomposing an obstinate eye movement desensitization target into smaller parts that we can do something with. Perhaps a good explanation also has to fit onto our working memory bandwidth. Since such reduction risks becoming an infinite regression, there must be some level at which we become satisfied with the explanation.

For our purposes here, I want an explanation that gives me some power, however limited, to predict what is going to happen next during treatment. It may only limit the possibilities, but sufficient that I know what to do next and can explain that to my patients. The explanation should be testable in the next step of research.

This explanation will be attempted in psychological terms and then in physiological terms, which we then try to connect. The physiological explanation is attempted in the next chapter. In this chapter, we explain eye movement desensitization as unloading an overloaded working memory. My explanation, and advice, on eye movement desensitization depends on the theory that post-traumatic strain disorder and similar illnesses are caused by saturation and strain of some limit in cognitive bandwidth. We need something with limited capacity to make this explanation work. This is the working memory and we attribute working memory overload as the proximal cause of chronic distress disorder. When we do eye movement therapy, or perhaps any effective psychological method, we are unloading working memory.

We require:

1. A definition of working memory.
2. A demonstration that anxiety and bad life experiences can affect working memory, or perhaps memory or cognition in general.
3. Evidence that eye movements can affect working memory.

9.3 WORKING MEMORY HAS A LIMITED CAPACITY

We recall that memory can be divided into various parts, initially long-term memory and short-term memory. Working memory is a better term for short-term memory, since this is where we do our thinking. Various definitions of working memory and similar things such as attention are available. All such definitions turn on the idea of limited capacity [110]. The limited capacity for immediate remembering was first noted in the 19th century [111]. When subjects were required to memorize items such as words, syllables or numbers, their performance deteriorated at around seven items. In 1887, London schoolchildren required to memorize syllables, numbers or words failed at around seven, eight or nine items [112]. This was considered to be the memory span, defining what could be held in memory at one time.

In 1956, Miller published his famous review, observing that seven was a common number found in cognitive and memory research [113]. This value was given as seven plus or minus two. That is, between five and nine but mostly seven. Seven often appears in psychological data. Seven might be a constant value for psychology in the way that other sciences have constant values [114]. Introductory textbooks often have lists of sevens. For example, the normal musical scale has seven intervals between eight notes. Another example is the organisation of a dictionary. Words in a dictionary are defined by words progressively simpler and more concrete, down to a base layer of words called atomic words. Analysis of English-language dictionaries from top-level abstract words to atomic words shows that they have seven layers [115].

The units of the seven were referred to as 'chunks'. A chunk is a piece of information that makes sense to the holder of that information. In laboratory experiments, it might be a word or number. In the real world, it might be something else, but difficult to define outside of controlled laboratories. More information can be included in the chunks with practice, repetition and skill. Expertise in a particular field is expressed as larger chunks, or perhaps as a hierarchical arrangement of chunks. Miller included images as possible chunks. The premise of the working memory explanation of eye movement therapy is that the flashbacks or distress images are chunks. They may be episodes (single events) or may be semantic memories. This means that similar events merged into one memory chunk because they share a similar meaning.

One definition of working memory is that it is that part of our memory that we are aware of using. It is the thinking space of the brain. We can use various metaphors or models for working memory. It may be a limitation of space, time, energy expenditure or physical capacity in some way. It might be that part of the long-term memory we switch on at one time, for a particular task [116].

In this explanation, working memory is an emergent property of attention, directed at any relevant memory network. We could say that attention is the function that turns on different parts of the regular memory network to varying extents [117]. That part of the long-term memory illuminated by the attention searchlight is working memory. In working memory, only one thing can be illuminated directly, but other items are still in the light to varying extents. This is because of some physical constraint in the system.

One idea that works well here is that working memory is the limit on the capacity of brain cells to communicate with each other. This is a limitation in the bandwidth of neuron membranes or axons. Such an explanation does not require working memory to be in one place in the brain. Instead, it emerges due to a limitation of the brain in normal use.

We can divide working memory into three parts:

1. The one-item focus of attention, the most activated part of long-term memory. Attention here lights up the thing in working memory that we want to use, or are instructing the patient to use.
2. The second region of access, containing three to five items. Laboratory tasks with strict definitions and methods, such as presenting visual stimuli and preventing rehearsal, reduce the number to four, plus or minus one [118].
3. The basal part of long-term memory, holding all the information relevant to a task, which is kept illuminated by rehearsal and reminders. This is the seven, plus or minus two, chunk of information.

9.4 CHASING THE SEVEN

This is my own observation of eye movement desensitization. Early in my experience with eye movement desensitization, it became apparent that the number of flashbacks or other distress images was limited. The impression was that it was limited to seven on average. I concluded that, like George Miller, I was being haunted by the number seven, or at least five to nine.

A retrospective count of 400 cases showed an average of 5.5 images [119]. After a retrospective observation, we should make a prospective prediction and then test it. The prediction was that the average number of distress images in a series of eye movement desensitization cases would tend to seven, plus or minus two. In the Genito-Urinary Medicine Clinic, patients were entered into a prospective case series, until 50 had completed treatment. Most were female sexual assault victims. The mean was 7.6 and both the median and mode were 7.0. Two other retrospective series also tended to seven [120].

Distribution of Images

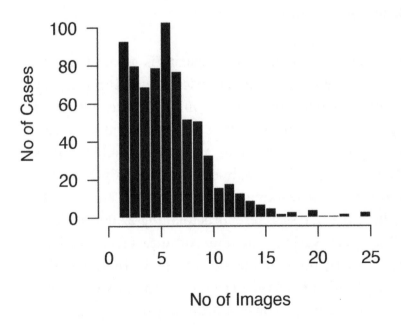

Fig 1.

Figure 1 is a histogram plot of all 722 cases for which I recorded a flashback number. This includes those who did not complete treatment but probably benefited from it (in my judgement) and then dropped out. The mean is 6.4, median is 6.0 and node is 6.0. The value falls off rapidly after seven. To express this with caution, this might be a signal from the working memory limit. This inspired the explanation given in this chapter and the advice in Chapter 8. This observation of a flashback horizon depends on the way eye movement therapy is performed, but that is the subject of this whole work.

9.5 ANXIETY AND TRAUMA DEFICITS IN WORKING MEMORY

We can claim that low memory capacity is associated with anxiety. This might mean that restricted working memory might cause anxiety or anxiety might cause restricted working memory. A meta-analysis is a statistical summary and investigation of research in a particular subject. It is an analysis of all previous analyses. A meta-analysis for the association between working memory capacity and anxiety issues collected 177 research reports totalling 22,000 subjects [121]. There are various methods of measuring working memory capacity, both simple and complex. There are also different methods of measuring or inducing anxiety, stress and worry. There was a consistent finding that high anxiety was associated with low working memory capacity, across different methods of measuring capacity and anxiety.

Another analysis of the structure of intelligence quotient (IQ) tasks, which used data collected from a website, collected results from 44,600 subjects. This showed that more anxious subjects performed worse on most tests, including working memory tests [122]. Another meta-analysis showed that cognitive deficits, including working memory issues, are associated with post-traumatic stress disorder [123]. In this report, data from 60 studies on 4000 subjects with post-traumatic stress disorder or trauma exposure, and including healthy controls, were combined. Post-traumatic stress disorder was associated with problems with working memory, attention, executive function, verbal learning and memory, visual learning and memory, and several other areas. These deficits were larger in respondents seeking treatment.

I want to claim here that restricted or over-loaded working memory causes anxiety, since that claim implies that unloading working memory will reduce anxiety. However, a correlation does not prove that low working memory capacity causes anxiety or vice versa. However, when people volunteer themselves into a situation that causes fear and anxiety, then any consequent reduction in working memory capacity shows causation. The working memory capacity of parachutists was measured in a plane before they jumped and after they had landed. As a control, working memory was measured on the ground on days when no jumps were scheduled. Working memory was lower in the plane before jumping. After landing, experienced parachutists recovered capacity while novice jumpers did not [124].

We can say that working memory capacity is reduced under anxiety or post-traumatic stress disorder. Elsewhere I say 'overloaded', which is near enough the same thing. My first reason for asserting that working memory is part of the explanation for the eye movement effect is the clinical observation that a blocked treatment will generally run again if the load on a patient's working memory or attention is reduced by decomposition. The second is the average of seven limit discussed above. The third is the evidence cited above. However, we should note that laboratory tests show that social anxiety correlates with high working memory capacity [125]. This is an unhelpful anomaly, especially since I recommend eye movement treatment for social anxiety elsewhere. Is there other support for the relation between working memory size, anxiety and eye movements?

9.6 EYE MOVEMENTS AFFECT WORKING MEMORY

Laboratory evidence shows movements can interfere with a visual working memory task, indicating that something is shared between them. Visual working memory, and the images held there, use the same control systems as voluntary eye movements. Subjects who made voluntary eye movements to indicate spatial locations showed reduced working memory performance on spatial tasks [126].

There is a link between visual working memory, attention and eye movements. Laboratory research shows that the eyes will move to a location where the attention has been directed in the absence of the actual object [127]. Attention, in the sense of a resource, is allocated to targets of possible eye movements.

It can be shown that the eye movements will react in the same way to remembered stimuli as they do to actual stimuli. Remembering a location may be equivalent to programming the oculomotor system to watch that location. Asking a patient to focus on an object in attention and artificially moving the eyes could disrupt this oculomotor program in some way.

9.7 WHY WE SHOULD LIKE THIS IDEA

The explanation that we are unloading overloaded working memory is helpful for these reasons:

1. The idea that we need to empty, or unload, a restricted working memory space, or bandwidth, enables clinical decisions. Most of the advice in Chapter 8 is based on this premise. For example, during treatment, distress may increase or fail to decrease. At this point, the toxic image exceeds the available memory processing bandwidth. One solution is to reduce the amount of information in the bandwidth. If the flashback is progressively reduced in some way, then the memory bandwidth frees up and the desensitization will start flowing again. By analogy, if we fail to pass a thread through the eye of the needle, we try smaller threads until it goes through.

2. A flashback that fails to change and does not yield to the above advice can be passed by. Work on easier flashbacks will clear the working memory bandwidth around the awkward one. This will either allow another attempt at treatment that may work or allow the decision that that issue is not eligible for treatment.

3. This liberated bandwidth enables further synergistic progress. We can now explain the cognitive and emotional change caused by the procedure. As memory bandwidth is liberated, the patient becomes progressively more able to think rationally. Distress is reduced to zero, or that level permitted by circumstances.

4. The observation of a limit to flashbacks gives us a diagnostic boundary that limits eye movement desensitization. If the patient fails to improve with eye movement desensitization above a certain number of flashbacks, then consider if it is wise to carry on. Elsewhere, it was reported that the average number of flashbacks or images is seven. About 98% of patients will report 14 or 15 or fewer distress images. Therefore, let us set this number at 15. Above this score, we will continue eye movement desensitization with a child sexual abuse patient with panic attacks, for example. However, we should watch to see if such a patient has treatment-resistant depression or a personality disorder that requires a change of method or advice from colleagues.

5. This idea of overloaded working memory is an explanation for the patient. Chronic distress, or strain, feels much like an overload. A script for explaining this is given at the end of this chapter.

6. Patients may enquire if they should stop, continue or proceed to other psychological therapy methods. If eye movement desensitization unloads an overloaded working memory, we can advise them that they could choose to continue with another method when they have a clean working memory. If eye movement desensitization has

been completed on all distress triggers, as advocated here, this should not be necessary, but it is the patient's choice.

7. Many patients will report serious bad life events or long histories of domestic abuse. The knowledge that the number of flashbacks is limited to seven enables the therapist and the patient to define the task. It also avoids the therapeutic nihilism these patients often attract.

8. The working memory explanation allows for natural recovery in people we do not see in clinics. Some victims sort out their own bandwidth, presumably the same way the rest of us do.

9. Unloading an overloaded working memory is the form of resource installation advocated here. The resource we are installing is working memory capacity or bandwidth. Accepting this permits the minimalist and utilitarian approach advocated here for the assessment and treatment method.

10. There are many things that cannot be sorted by moving the patient's eyes from side to side. I commonly say to my patients that eye movement desensitization is only memory repair, not moral reconciliation. It does not make bad things good, or make bad people good. It just repairs some of the damage. However, a clean working memory may empower the patient to deal with these things.

11. In the next chapter, I compare artificial eye movements to the various eye movements observed in sleep. However, there are methods of eye movement desensitization that use other methods of sensory stimulation or taxing working memory. We need a way of accounting for these methods. The working memory explanation is consistent with the effect of these other methods.

9.8 REVERSE LEARNING

It is initially confusing that we do not have to use eye movements to do 'eye movement' desensitization. We will have to continue to call it that until a less confusing name is found. I suggest 'neural network desensitization'. There are different methods and I listed auditory and tactile in the last chapter. No doubt others will be found.

Reverse learning is a model of memory consolidation during rapid eye movement sleep. It is derived from computer models of brain function called neural networks. Such models represent information held in nerve cells as a number, which represents the activation or energy level of the cell. Neural network theory enables mathematical and computed models of psychological phenomena which are testable. The theory of reverse learning was published in 1986 by Crick & Mitchison [128]. It may explain, or at least model, what happens with artificial eye movements. The information for different memories can overlap at a given location in the neural network, depending on the degree of association between those memories. Such common points, or nodes, will be where the memories have a common element. For our purposes, a node is a mathematical model of a group of neurons with a common property, such as common information. In the real brain, such a node may hold all the distress memories linked by a common element, such as an image of the event or the villain or bad thoughts such as loss of control or self-blame. A node has a limited capacity like any physical system. Excess information, represented by activity or energy, will overload this node. When this overflow happens, the wrong associations will form between information at other nodes not logically connected. The neural net will then behave pathologically, perhaps producing a confused output of different memories, or repeatedly showing it's owner the overloaded information.

Such bad memories are called parasitic memories, because they occupy the node at the expense of normal memories, like a cuckoo chick in the nest of a willow warbler. We can reasonably equate distress flashbacks with parasitic memories. How should we fix this problem? Memory could be cleared by resetting all nodes to zero, but this would cause zero memory, so that is not biologically plausible.

A method is required that preserves or consolidates new memories and forgets those that are old, redundant or parasitic. In our context, it is the unwanted emotional component of the memory that overloads the nodes, rather than the dry facts, and which needs to be lost. Neural network simulations show that such overloading can be lost by switching off the input and output channels of the net and sending pulses of activation through the system. These spikes of energy do not code for any memories because no input is synchronized with them.

This neural network model shows that it is possible to switch off the input and output of the neural network and subject it to a series of non-specific activations. This is reverse learning. Here is a simpler model of this model. Imagine a tray of sand, where the layer of sand is flat. The energy level of the sand grains is equal because all are at the same level. The sand can also exist in a second state where it has been scooped into a pile. In the second state, the energy levels of the sand grains differ, since they are at different physical levels. How do we return the sand to its original state? We could tap the tray with a hammer, sending a similar energy pulse into each grain of sand regardless of its position in the pile. The pulse is not specific to the energy level of the sand grains. This shakedown would return the sand to the first state.

How does reverse learning help us?

Assume that the total capacity of each node is the capacity of working memory. Then we have a link between reverse learning and the working memory explanation. Overloaded working memory is equivalent to an overloaded node. It is then reasonable and helpful to imagine that the distress score is a proxy for the activation or energy in the strained node. At zero, the index node would be equivalent to it's neighbouring nodes. The network is in equilibrium. At higher scores, the node becomes a bad neighbour. The network becomes strained around it and distress ensues.

This gives us a direct, if abstract, understanding of what we are doing when we move our eyes or similar. This takes us into the next chapter, where I consider artificial and natural eye movements. When does the brain close off it's input and output and send energy spikes through itself? Obviously, when it is asleep. The likely candidate for the energy spikes is identified in Chapter 10. This explanation is consistent with other methods of sensory stimulation. Eye movements might be the best way to hijack the reverse learning machine, but not the only way.

There is a general point here concerning the usefulness of neural network theory. It provides a way to a unified theory of psychology [129]. It provides an understanding of post-traumatic stress disorder and other forms of chronic distress, and of eye movement therapy that evades the risks of narrative accounts. The idea is that nodes in a network hold information, transmit it to other nodes or may be unable to transmit it to others because they are overloaded.

The patient is distressed when this bandwidth is jammed. This makes sense of much of what we seek to understand here. For example, a flashback that fails to desensitize is an overloaded node that is stuck. One solution is to move to another flashback that shares or is connected to the stuck node. Reducing the second flashback may siphon off some of the stuck activation (i.e. distress or strain) from the first.

9.9 EXPLAINING TO THE PATIENT

Our memory is divided into two parts. The first is long-term memory, where we keep all our information. The second is short-term memory. This is where we do our thinking and is better called working memory. The words I am saying right now are floating round in the air, going through your ears and into the working memory in your brain, where you understand the meaning of them. The problem with working memory is that it has only a limited capacity. In general, it can handle only about seven things at once. When people have post-traumatic stress disorder (or whatever the issue is) it is caused by overloaded working memory.

So if you own three flashbacks and are being reminded of them all the time, then you can think about only four other things. This is why people have memory loss and concentration problems and do not see other risks approaching.

10. MOVING EYES

10.1 WHAT HAPPENS WHEN THE EYES MOVE?

Changes in a well-conducted eye movement therapy session can happen fast. This means something physiological is happening. What happens when we ask someone to move their eyes artificially? If we pursue the nerve signals caused by the movement of the target from the fovea through the network of visual and brain science reports, we end up with the whole brain. We are also not restricted to the visual system in eye movement desensitization. In this chapter, I will try to indicate some elements of a physiological explanation. Specifically, is our method artificial dreaming? Bear with me here if I skim over issues, neglect possibilities or lose whole visual pathways. We have only 20 or so pages to sketch physiological possibilities and whole books have been written to explain how the brain works or just on eye movements. We must now record further limitations of our explanation, numbered consecutively from the last chapter. This gives us a total of 20 caveats as boundaries to our attempt to explain.

14. We can agree that patients receiving eye movement therapy are awake. If we are considering artificial dreaming as an explanation, we must find a way to compare phenomena in the awake brain with events in the asleep brain. If this phenomena is not present in the awake brain, then we are arguing by analogy, not homology. We must be modulating those day phenomena, rather than some night phenomena. There is an escape clause from this caveat, which is discussed below.

15. Although electrical signals are discussed below as a way of interpreting events in the brain, we should also allow that the brain has mechanical, and may have quantum mechanical, methods of signalling [130,131]. Neither are considered here. Also, we do not have a complete understanding of how nerve cells communicate. Ordinary cells – that is, not nerve cells – also communicate by bioelectricity, which is not understood well.

16. Changes in memory during sleep are referred to as memory consolidation, but this is not what we require from eye movement desensitization. What we require from eye movement desensitization is desensitization, at the risk of stating the obvious. In fact, memory consolidation is the problem, not the solution, since distress memories can be consolidated without reducing distress.

17. Below we consider the two stages of sleep, each of which can be further subdivided. Other distinctions are procedural or declarative memory, with declarative divided into episodic or semantic. There is also remembering, consolidating and encoding memory information. This is too many combinations to deal with here. I will not strive to ascribe particular functions to particular sleep stages in my attempt below to discover if eye movement desensitization mimics any particular sleep function.

18. So much is reported about the brain and its workings that one could probably find a connection between any part or function you wanted to. Caution is required about any such conclusions.

19. The function of most brain signals is obscure. Some correlations are known with memory changes. However, there is a problem at an abstract level. Just because we talk in terms of emotion, memory or anxiety does not mean the brain works with those concepts. This is similar to the problem with phrenology in the 19th century. Personality characters were attributed to variations in the shape of the skull. We now know this to be wrong. It might be a similar error to attribute memory change to a brain signal.

20. How do we explain brain action anyway? The attempt at explanation made below depends on identifying possible brain phenomena that might cause desensitization. If we can link these phenomena to eye movements, we can speculate if artificial eye movements might hijack the same phenomena. Is this the right method of explanation? It is premised on the locationist argument. This assumes that

phenomena such as fear or anxiety, or perhaps good and bad affect, are located in a specific part of the brain, or at least depend on that part of the brain. There is an assumption that we can explain our problem by finding the place in the brain where desensitization happens. Discovering where it happens in the brain equals discovering how it happens in the brain. It can be assumed that such locationist arguments are convincing and considered to trump other methods of explanation. This may not be true. There might be larger networks that have more abstract functions. If so, a claim that artificial eye movements simulate function X in location Y, where we might intercept and destroy bad emotions, may not work. If, as I suspect at the end of the chapter, desensitization happens everywhere in the brain, then this locationist argument loses most of its power of explanation.

10.2 IS EYE MOVEMENT DESENSITIZATION ARTIFICIAL DREAMING?

Perhaps eye movement therapy is artificial rapid eye movement sleep. Dreaming is associated with rapid eye movement sleep and maybe this indicates memory consolidation. There is an intuitive idea that rapid eye movements in dreams are scanning images and acting on them in some way. Perhaps artificial eye movements disrupt mental images. I once tried out the idea that artificial eye movements might affect images using a model called reverse learning [132]. In the last chapter, we noted that the theory or model of reverse learning was helpful as part of this explanation. Computer models of artificial neural networks show that overloaded nodes in the network can contain pathological information.

This problem can be fixed by closing off the input and output of the network and then applying a random activation signal to the network. This shakes down the network into a healthy state, in which bad information, defined by overloading, is discarded, but pre-existing good information is preserved. If we look at a real brain, what happens that looks like this? The brain when asleep, when input and output are closed off, or at least reduced. In particular, rapid eye movement sleep, when ponto-geniculo-occipital spikes travel through the brain. These nerve impulses start in the pons, in the brainstem. The four optical motor nerves go to the pons. Perhaps moving eyes artificially sends a signal to the pons, which triggers ponto-geniculo-occipital spikes. I like this idea, but it is not as simple as this. I will discuss the original basis for this notion, what problems arise and if these issues can be mitigated.

10.3 SLEEP STAGES

Rapid eye movement sleep is one of two stages in human sleep. Our eyes move when we are asleep. In sleep time, there are two different types of eye movements: rapid and slow. Sleep is divided into two primary stages: rapid eye movement sleep (REM) and non-rapid eye movement sleep (NREM). Rapid eye movements occur in, and define, rapid eye movement sleep. Sleep starts in the non-rapid eye movement stage and then progresses to the rapid eye movement stage (NREM → REM). During a night of normal sleep, we alternate between rapid eye movement sleep and non-rapid eye movement sleep in four cycles [133].

The non-rapid eye movement sleep stage is further divided into three secondary stages ($N1$ → $N2$ → $N3$). These secondary stages are defined by the depth of sleep and other physiological parameters, which we will not consider further. Stage $N1$ is somnolence – sleepy, but not quite asleep yet. Stage $N2$ is light sleep. Stage $N3$ is deep sleep and also slow wave sleep. This is considered further below. The second sort of sleep eye movements, slow eye movements, do not define non-rapid eye movement sleep or slow wave sleep (delta waves). Slow eye movements occur throughout all stages, including rapid eye movement sleep. Being awake is considered another stage, which completes the classification. In normal, non-pathological sleep, rapid eye movement sleep always occurs between periods of non-rapid eye movement sleep. A sleep cycle is a sequence of sleep stages.

$$\text{NREM } [N1 \rightarrow N2 \rightarrow N3] \rightarrow \text{REM}$$

Each cycle lasts about 90 minutes and there are four cycles a night. The share of rapid eye movement sleep increases towards the end. Rapid eye movement sleep can be further divided into two microstates called phasic and tonic. This is considered below.

10.4 WHY DO WE HAVE RAPID EYE MOVEMENT SLEEP?

Sleep, and in particular rapid eye movement sleep, shows much of the properties we need to explain eye movement desensitization [134]. Sleep loss and disruption is associated with psychiatric illness and emotional disorder. Experimental sleep deprivation increases stress, anxiety, anger and impulsive behaviour in laboratory tests. Rapid eye movement sleep consolidates fear memories, improving later discrimination between fear and non-fear-causing stimuli. It also increases extinction of fear memories that experience shows are no longer required. It may decrease the emotional load of a memory, but keep the factual part. This is required to know the dangerous thing, but not overreact to or misidentify the danger trigger.

Perhaps artificial eye movements simulate or mimic this process. What is it that we are simulating? Any enquiry after the function, or rather functions, of rapid eye movement sleep is a subset of enquiry about all the sleep stages. Functions such as reducing the emotional content of memories might be part of memory consolidation and may occur during sleep stages.

We will agree, without going into it too much here, that sleep consolidates memory. Relative to wakefulness, sleep is good for memories. What is consolidation? Memories must be acquired and encoded in the neurons while we are awake, and then also retrieved while awake. To be useful, similar memories must attract each other, and become integrated or connected and remain so for as long as we require them.

Irrelevant information must be discarded. In this way, related episodic memories become one semantic memory.

This process of integration is called consolidation. A consolidated memory trace is stronger in the sense that it is remembered better, or is more resistant to forgetting. We can assume that such consolidation should happen when the animal is asleep and the memory information is not required. However, this area is difficult to pin down because so many factors interact. There is some evidence that consolidation occurs when we are awake [135–137].

Consolidation may not supply us with all the explanation we require because distress memories and images can be consolidated, or perhaps inadequately consolidated, while still toxic. We require that memories are relieved of toxic emotional content, which we call desensitization.

Sleep disturbance is associated with post-traumatic stress disorder and anxiety and has been shown to precede it after a bad life event [138]. Increased eye movements per minute in rapid eye movement sleep predict post-traumatic stress disorder. Rapid eye movement sleep fragmentation after a bad event also predicts post-traumatic stress disorder [139].

What are ponto-geniculo-occipital spikes?

Ponto-geniculo-occipital spikes are a series of nerve impulses, or trains of spikes. The acronym is PGO. They are sometimes referred to as 'PGO waves', but 'wave' is used in the sense of a series of spikes. I am not using that word here to avoid confusion with waves in the sense of the oscillations observed by electroencephalography. These spike trains are detected with electrodes inserted into the brain of a laboratory animal, usually a cat. They occur maximally in the pons (in the brainstem), the lateral geniculate nucleus (underneath the centre of the brain) and the occipital lobes (at the back of the brain). They occur during rapid eye movement sleep [140,141]. These signals can also be detected in non-rapid eye movement sleep and when awake. Rapid eye movement sleep deprivation increases subsequent ponto-geniculo-occipital spike trains.

Assume the spikes and rapid eye movement sleep are related. To connect both, we could assert that rapid eye movements are a leakage of ponto-geniculo-occipital spike trains down the visual motor nerves to the eye muscles. If we do this, then we are assuming that the eye moments in sleep do not have a primary function. To employ the correct word, sleep rapid eye movements are an epiphenomenon of ponto-geniculo-occipital spikes. This is in the context of our explanation. Other functions are attributed to rapid eye movement sleep but we will not consider them here.

Under laboratory conditions, sleep eye movements can be decreased with repeated low-frequency auditory tones [142]. This is associated with an increased electroencephalography signal, which possibly indicates decreased ponto-geniculo-occipital spikes, and decreased dream imagery reports. This shows that an external stimulus, which resembles that used in auditory eye movement desensitization, can affect ponto-geniculo-occipital spikes.

What are the visual motor nerves?

The relevant motor nerves are the oculomotor, trochlear and abducens cranial nerves. The ophthalmic nerve may also have motor functions. There are twelve cranial nerves. They emerge from the cranium, which is the part of the skull that houses the brain. Cranial nerves are distinct from other nerves, which originate in the spinal chord. Eleven cranial nerves carry sensory and motor signals for the head, and the vagus nerve wanders down below the neck to do interesting things with other organs. The nerves that matter here are the five connected to the eyes:

1. **The optic nerve**. This is a sensory nerve that connects the retina of the eye with the lateral geniculate nucleus, which is below the centre of the brain. This nerve sends signals of an image, and the movements of that image, to the brain.

2. **The oculomotor nerve**. This nerve, and the next two below, are the three motor nerves, whose function is to contract certain muscles to move the eyes. The oculomotor nerve is busy. It contracts four out of the six muscles outside the eyeball, making the eye move up, down or sideways. It moves the upper eyelid up, which is necessary when looking up. It contracts muscles inside the eye that accommodate to changes in light. It originates in the oculomotor nuclear complex in the midbrain.

3. **The trochlear nerve.** This contracts one muscle outside the eye that moves the eye inwards and downwards. It originates in the trochlear nucleus in the midbrain. When it leaves the midbrain, it crosses over, so that the nerve

originating from the right side goes to the left eye and vice versa.

4. **The abducens nerve.** This controls one muscle that moves the eye from side to side. If we move our eyes from side to side artificially, we must be exploiting the abducens nerve mostly and the oculomotor and trochlear nerves to a lesser extent. The abducens nerve originates from the abducens nucleus in the pontine tegmentum. It is convenient for our purposes that the pontine tegmentum is active during rapid eye movement sleep and presumably drives it. This structure is part of the pons, which is in the brainstem below the midbrain.

5. **The ophthalmic branch of the trigeminal nerve.** The trigeminal nerve provides motor and sensory supply to the face. It has three branches, and today ours is the ophthalmic nerve. It signals touch, pain, temperature and proprioception from the eye and orbit to the brain.

Do humans have ponto-geniculo-occipital spikes?

The short answer is yes, we do. If cat brains have PGO spikes, then primate and human brains do. Mammalian brains are likely to be similar, given the evolutionary history discussed in Chapter 11. However, it is good biology to be cautious about direct homology between species. Things can change over time and there is a lot of time to be allowed for. In humans, electrodes can be implanted in the brains of patients for clinical reasons. For example, electrodes are used for deep brain stimulation in patients with Parkinson's disease. They are not put on the track of any passing ponto-geniculo-occipital spike trains, but we may see them passing if they are implanted in the thalamus, which is above the pons and the brainstem. Using this method, signals can be detected in human rapid eye movement sleep that are probably ponto-geniculo-occipital trains [143,144]. Another deep electrode study observed that neurons in the medial temporal lobe and neocortex showed signals during rapid eye movements when both asleep and awake that were transient biphasic nerve spike trains that looked like ponto-geniculo-occipital trains [145]. This signal reduced before the rapid eye movements and increased after them.

What causes ponto-geniculo-occipital spikes?

These nerve spikes originate in the pons, which is part of the brainstem. Certain neurons there can act as a signal generator. Within the pons, one area where this signal generation takes place is the pontine tegmentum, where the abducens oculomotor nerve originates. External sensory stimuli can affect ponto-geniculo-occipital spikes. A loudspeaker tone can trigger spikes in the lateral geniculate nucleus and occipital lobes [146].

Can we say that artificial eye movements trigger ponto-geniculo-occipital spikes?

'Not yet' is the best answer. We can speculate the case that moving the patient's eyes artificially might cause something similar to ponto-geniculo-occipital spikes. Moving the eyes could cause a signal in the three motor nerves that go from the eye muscle to the brainstem. Feedback through motor nerves is called proprioception, which is the sense of the position and movement of the body. This sense is signalled by certain sensory organs in the muscles. The oculomotor muscles have organs that detect movement and this outflowing, or afferent, nerve signal is transmitted through the oculomotor nerves to the brain. In physiological studies of experimental animals, these signals can be detected in certain areas of the brain [147]. For our purposes, note that this includes the brainstem, the lateral geniculate nucleus and the visual cortex.

In one of the few references to laboratory animal reports that I use, there is a helpful observation in rats [148]. Rodents do not quite have ponto-geniculo-occipital spikes. They have P-waves, which have been observed only in the rat pons, and not in the lateral geniculate nucleus. Rats can be trained to fear a laboratory enclosure with electric shocks to the foot. The amount of fear is measured by the proportion of freezing behaviour. The fear reduces or extinguishes if the rat is left alone in the enclosure without any human oppression. P-waves were counted as waves per minute of sleep time during a six-hour sleep/awake observation time after training. This value is called the 'density', although I think 'frequency' might be a better word. The P-wave density increased in the first three hours of the six-hour sleep cycle after the extinction of fear. The more freezing behaviour, the higher the P-wave density. The correlation between fear behaviour and P-wave frequency was 0.95, which is high for behavioural data. This looks like P-waves are associated with fear extinction. However, it does not show that P-waves cause fear extinction.

Does this explanation work?

The attempt at comparing eye movement desensitization with rapid eye movement sleep must be the route to explanation, but it attracts a list of seven problems.

Problem 1. Some caution is indicated in concluding that the function of rapid eye movement is simply sorting out bad memories or emotions. Perhaps rapid eye movements in sleep are an epiphenomenon – that is, a side effect of some other primary event or function. For example, men in rapid eye movement sleep experience activity of the penis that does not relate to sexual dreams. We would not conclude that the function of rapid eye movement sleep is male penis activity.

Problem 2. Newborns have up to eight hours of rapid eye movement sleep each day, before collecting any bad life events. Rapid eye movements also occur before birth. People with lifelong blindness and no visual dreams have rapid eye movement sleep [149]. This implies that rapid eye movements in sleep are not caused or preceded by, or may have reasons other than, visual experience.

Problem 3. Large numbers of people have their rapid eye movement sleep disrupted and reduced by both depression and anti-depressant medication [150]. If memory consolidation was the exclusive function of rapid eye movement sleep then we should conclude that these patients are probably not consolidating memories. However, they survive, or at least get by, so loss of rapid eye movement sleep is not fatal, or essential for memory consolidation.

Problem 4. Not many rapid eye movements happen in rapid eye movement sleep. The word 'rapid' applies to the speed of movement, not the frequency of the events. Rapid eye movements do not appear in about 80% of rapid eye movement sleep time. This is the distinction between phasic and tonic microstates, considered further below. So, if the eye movements are doing something, they are not very busy.

Problem 5. Dreams can be recorded in non-rapid eye movement sleep. Dreaming was once considered to happen only during rapid eye movement sleep. Subjects woken in this phase report dreams and their electroencephalography signals are similar to those in waking. However, when subjects are asked the right question, mental activity is reported in non-rapid eye movement sleep. We dream in all stages of sleep [151,152]. We cannot cite dreams to support a comparison of rapid eye movement sleep and eye movement desensitization.

Problem 6. The sixth problem is slow eye movements. These happen in all stages of sleep, but their frequency decreases across the secondary stages of non-rapid eye movement sleep and then it increases again in the rapid eye movement stage [153]. The percentage of time in each stage that slow eye movements are observed is given below, with the rapid eye movement stage shown at the beginning of the sequence:

REM (43%) → NREM [N 1 (54%) → N 2 (21%) → N 3 (10%)]

Therefore, most slow eye movements happen in the first stage of non-rapid eye movement sleep (N 1) and in the rapid eye movement sleep stage. The slow eye movements are at a minimum in stage three (N 3), when slow delta waves (and spindles) are at a maximum (delta waves and spindles are discussed below).

I cannot find any report that describes a physiological basis or function for slow eye movements in the same way that we might link ponto-geniculo-occipital trains to rapid eye movements (in humans). However, slow eye movements must result from activity in the visual system. The issue is that we cannot exclude slow eye movements in sleep from our explanation. The only reason to privilege rapid eye movements was the association with dreaming and then linking that to emotional memory consolidation. However, if slow eye movements happen during rapid eye movement sleep, then they have an equal right to be linked with dreaming.

We cannot sustain a privileged link between rapid eye movements and dreaming or equate dreaming with desensitizing toxic memories. It follows that we must be cautious about any simple comparison of eye movement desensitization with rapid eye movement sleep. Perhaps a brain function that preferably runs in rapid eye movement sleep time can also run in awake time, even though this may not be optimum. How is this possible if we use the premise that the function of rapid eye movement is to consolidate, or desensitize, toxic memories?

One solution is that it is not the function of rapid eye movement sleep to sort out memories. Perhaps we must look back 200 million years, not 20 or 200 years, to understand the functions of sleep stages. There is a useful idea that the origin of sleep and sleep stages is located in hundreds of millions of years of evolutionary history ('deep time'). Sleep stages were not caused by the need for memory consolidation, desensitization or any contemporary concern. Sleep stages may have originated in other behavioural and physiological contingencies.

This excuses us from requiring that contemporary sleep stages have evolved for some specific or exclusive purpose, such as memory consolidation. The consequence of this is that we need not worry too much about contradictory evidence for any particular current function of rapid eye movement sleep or any other sleep stage. This mitigates the problem that our initial comparison between eye movement desensitization and rapid eye movement sleep suffers from – the disadvantage that one happens when awake and the other when asleep. Further discussion of this issue is relegated to Chapter 11.

Problem 7. Any comparison of eye movement desensitization to rapid eye movement sleep is inadequate by itself because more than one thing must be happening when we move our, or the patient's, eyes.

10.5 WHAT ELSE HAPPENS WHEN THE EYES MOVE?

As you read this, the image of the words on this line is now travelling from your eyes down the optic nerve to the lateral geniculate nucleus, to the visual cortex, and onto the other 12 topographically organized visual areas in the brain. These areas are connected to other parts of the brain, some of which send instructions to the eye muscles, telling your eyes to move along this line. This focus of reading attention moves along the line, controlled by your understanding, progress and perhaps your agreement with our subject. A lot must be happening.

For our purposes here, there are two sorts of eye movement when awake [154,155]. Eye movements start when the target moves off the fovea. The fovea is that part of the retina with the highest resolution. If it were a camera sensor chip, it would have the smallest pixels. Visual acuity decreases if the target moves off the fovea. Smooth movements track a target slowly, keeping it on the fovea. Saccades are faster movements that catch up with the target when required or look elsewhere to acquire another target. Saccades cannot be distinguished in either shape or speed from rapid eye movements in sleep [145]. Smooth eye movements will retain the target on the fovea while saccades will place it there. Saccades are the catch-up when smooth movements are not fast enough and the target fails to stay on the fovea. When doing artificial eye movements, we are most likely to trigger smooth movements.

We need to describe what is happening in a patient's brain when the patient is not moving and looking at a visual field that is static except for our moving target. We must visit the larger problem of how the brain locates objects when the brain's owner is always moving. Because the owner is mobile, the location of an object's image on the retina does not determine where it is in space. However, we see a stable visual field. To achieve this stable perception, we need more information, which we pick up on the retina. For a brain's owner to locate an object in space so it can be touched, avoided or tracked, the brain must allow for movements.

There are two possible ways to do this [156]. The first is corollary discharge, in which the part of the brain that controls movement sends a copy of the motor signal to the visual part of the brain, which integrates it with the visual signal. This allows a predictive mapping of body movement. This signal is retinotropic – that is, centred on the position of the eye – and works rapidly and approximately. The corollary discharge signal is used in various areas of the brain, including the superior colliculus and frontal eye fields, to adjust signals from the retina. We can note that when we ask the patient to do eye movement desensitization there are no corollary discharges because we have instructed the patient to sit still.

The second mechanism is oculomotor proprioception [157]. Proprioception is the sense that signals the position and movement of the muscles. A proprioceptive signal is slower, but more accurate and craniotopic. The signal is calculated relative to the head position and the centre of the gaze when the subject is looking ahead. Proprioceptive sense organs are found in the muscles and tendons of the ocular muscles. These control eye movements and are controlled by the oculomotor nerves. These organs are the most likely source of proprioceptive feedback for eye position.

Nerve signals from eye position movements are found in parts of the brain that are relevant to our case, such as the superior colliculus, lateral geniculate nucleus, central thalamus, posterior parietal cortex (including areas with a visual function), and the frontal eye fields. A signal with eye movement information that is not from the retina can be detected in the visual cortex [158].

Anyway, we could chase visual signals all around the brain if we had the space and time, but we are stopping here. In the end, we are visual animals and many parts of our brains process visual information. Locating a signal to particular locations may not be the point. We could also get lost again in the brain if we attempted to locate other sensory signals, such as sound, which also have desensitization abilities. It must be true that the eye movement signal is received in many parts of the brain. Eye movement desensitization is not sensory-specific. Eye movements control auditory or other sense flashbacks. Auditory bleeps control visual flashbacks. The various interoceptive or physical sensations, from different body locations, can also be controlled. Perhaps we should look at signals from the whole brain for any useful clues to our problem.

10.6 WHAT IS SEEN WITH ELECTROENCEPHALOGRAPHY?

Neural activity in the brain can be detected on the surface of the head as electrical signals [159]. These signals are detected with electroencephalography (EEG). This is a large subject and here I list only some frequencies and give some examples of why we might be interested in these signals [160].

Electroencephalography is the recording of voltage fluctuations by electrodes on the surface of the head. A variation of this is to place the electrodes on the surface of the brain during surgery. The signal these electrodes receive is a summary or addition of the signals from the 80 billion neurons in the brain. If two spikes from two neurons arrive together at a third neuron, their power will add together and affect the third neuron that much more. If a third spike arrives a little later from a fourth neuron, it will have less effect on the third neuron. A larger number of spikes arriving at the third neuron at the same time will become a wave with a peak at the most common time of arrival. Imagine waves arriving at a beach, while you sit in the edge of the sea, watching them approach. If two or more arrive together, they may combine and go over your head. A third wave arriving later may go up only to your elbows.

When a large number of spikes arrive together, the amplitude, or power, is high and this is referred to as synchronization. If fewer arrive, the amplitude and power is lower, and these are desynchronized. A series of waves is an oscillation. The oscillations come in various frequency bands, from 0.05Hz to 600Hz. (Hz = hertz, defined as a change in a periodic event of one cycle per second. Hertz is the unit of frequency.) It is possible that there are frequencies above or below this range that cannot be detected by current methods and evade participation in our story.

One parameter that describes the wave is the amplitude, or height, of the wave. This is considered as a measure of the power contained in a wave. More power means a higher amplitude, which means more neurons are firing together. However, other events reduce the amplitude of an observed wave. It can vary due to other factors, such as anatomical differences, the conductivity of tissue (such as the bone of the skull), the presence of other charged molecules (such as proteins), cerebral blood flow, muscle activity, blood chemistry and carbon dioxide levels [161]. Surface electroencephalography does not see discrete signals from deeper brain structures. These electroencephalography frequencies may not have a causal role in brain actions. They may just be the top-down cumulative signal of other events. Possibly, these signals are the electrical ticks of the brain's clock, which is used to synchronize brain activity. Below we note five classes of waves and two other related observations.

1. Alpha (α) waves

These are mostly recorded in the occipital region at frequencies of between 8 and 12 Hz. The highest amplitude is over the posterior and occipital regions – that is, the visual cortex. The amplitude can be up to 50 microvolts and is maximal in a relaxed subject with closed eyes. With electrodes implanted in the brain, this signal can be detected in the occipital lobes and down to the lateral geniculate nucleus. Alpha waves disappear during sleep.

Alpha waves might be a candidate for a role in the eye movement desensitization story because they can be externally modified by a stimulus or task. Alpha waves decrease in power, indicating desynchronization, with a perceptual change, a decision or increased attention. It has been shown that switching a sound on and off can synchronize alpha waves in the visual cortex [162]. This results in increased amplitude. Perhaps the auditory version of eye movement treatment increases the amplitude of alpha waves.

2. Theta (Θ) waves

These are a regular oscillation with a sinusoidal shape, between 4 and 8 Hz [163]. This signal originates in the thalamus. Other centres in the brain synchronize or entrain these oscillations. Subjects who had experienced a trauma event were grouped into those who had developed post-traumatic stress disorder and those who had not [164]. Their theta waves were observed during rapid eye movement sleep. The patients who had not developed post-traumatic stress disorder had more theta wave power.

3. Gamma (Γ) waves

These are found at 30 to 100 Hz in the somatosensory cortex. They may indicate processes in local networks in the brain. Smooth and saccadic eye movements can increase the gamma power in certain brain regions, including the frontal eye field and the medial occipital gyrus, which is the location of the of the visual cortex [155].

4. Delta (Δ) waves

These are at 0.75 to 4 Hz. They appear in the third substage, slow wave sleep, of non-rapid eye movement sleep (N 3). Delta waves are associated with neuronal changes caused by activity or learning. One demonstration of this is that immobilizing an arm for 12 hours causes reduced performance on a simple reaching task. Electroencephalography of the relevant arm zone of the motor cortex during sleep shows reduced delta activity [166].

5. Spindles

These signals appear in non-rapid eye movement sleep, mostly in stage N 2 [167,168]. They are mostly seen in the thalamus, cortex and neocortex. The frequency is 12 to 14 Hz, decreasing to zero amplitude in one second or less. They occur in bursts of five to fifteen oscillations. Sleep spindles increase in density (or frequency) over the night. The occurrence of spindles can be positively related to improved memory test results and increased intelligence quotient scores. Perhaps eye movement therapy increases spindle frequency.

6. Global field synchronization of rapid eye movement sleep

The degree to which neuron spikes combine into the waves that comprise the electroencephalography signal is called coherence or synchronization. Global field synchronization is a similar measure, but combined over time. The value is the correlation between the signal in consecutive four-second time periods within each of the frequency bands given above. Since the signal originates in different places in the brain, a higher correlation value most likely indicates that those parts of the brain are synchronized. The different parts are working together [169].

There are three states of existence: awake, rapid eye movement sleep, and non-rapid eye movement sleep. Global field synchronization correlation is highest in rapid eye movement sleep, in all frequency bands, with two exceptions. There were higher values when spindles occurred and equal values in the theta band in both sleep states. Therefore, there is a high state of common brain activity in rapid eye movement sleep. This is helpful because we are basing our explanation of eye movement desensitization on this sleep state. I would like to know what happens to the global field synchronization value in the fourth state of existence, in which the awake patient sits still and the eyes are moved artificially.

7. Phasic and tonic rapid eye movement sleep

Another problem in enlisting rapid eye movement sleep in an explanation is that it has two parts. The phasic part is the actual eye movements, in between the tonic part where the eyes are still [170,171]. The brain is less responsive during phasic rapid eye movement sleep to sensory stimulation. Electroencephalography from surgical depth electrodes showed that the signal in certain brain areas in the phasic microstate was similar to that in waking when an image was shown, or during voluntary movement. The brain is more responsive in the tonic microstate.

There are differences in the electroencephalography amplitude at different frequencies. The tonic microstate showed higher power in alpha and beta bands. The phasic microstate showed higher power in the gamma and delta range. The high global field synchronization values found in rapid eye movement sleep can be located in the phasic part in the delta and theta range, and in the tonic part the beta band was higher. This indicates that different things are happening in each part of rapid eye movement sleep. The phasic events must be the best model for eye movement desensitization.

10.7 OBSERVED PHYSIOLOGICAL CHANGES

Considered here are some of the observed physiological changes found in eye movement desensitization [172]. Brain signals have been observed during eye movement desensitization [173]. Ten patients receiving eye movement desensitization were observed with electroencephalography during their first and last sessions. All distress triggers were desensitized to a score of zero. A script of their worst bad life events was used as a standard trigger. Signals were recorded with the patient at rest, listening to the script with eyes closed, before and after treatment.

Before treatment, the highest power signals were found in the prefrontal cortex and limbic regions. After treatment, the highest signal was found in the fusiform and visual cortex. Patients also had a higher power signal in the limbic area before treatment than the controls. Changes were found in all frequency bands analysed by brain site. The alpha and theta bands changed the most. The hippocampus is a part of the limbic system. The limbic system has been described as the location of emotional processing. The fusiform area specializes in certain stimuli, notably faces. It may be that the movement of the synchronized signal peak from the emotional part of the brain to the non-emotional sensory areas is related to a decrease of the bad emotion due to treatment. However, we are being cautious about matching psychology to physiology using electroencephalography.

Physiological measurements have been taken during eye movement sessions [174]. Thirteen patients were observed during treatment [174]. Their heart rate decreased progressively over the sets of eye movements. Their breathing frequency also decreased, as did their skin conductance. This indicates a decrease in activity in the sympathetic nervous system, which is that part of the nervous system that increases the ability of the body to cope with stress stimuli.

Some physiological observations were made on Swedish train drivers who had seen people jump in front of their train or had seen people assaulted [175]. The train drivers were divided into patients with post-traumatic stress disorder and a control group. Cerebral blood flow was measured using a brain scan. The patients had increased blood flow in certain parts of the brain before eye movement desensitization treatment. Treatment reduced the blood flow to levels similar to those of the controls. The brain areas include the visual cortex and the hippocampus.

There is evidence for a change in the volume of parts of the brain after eye movement therapy. An increase in hippocampal volume and a decrease in thalamus volume was observed in treated patients compared with untreated healthy control subjects [176]. These patients had a smaller hippocampus volume before treatment. Recall from the second chapter that a small hippocampal volume is a risk factor for post-traumatic stress disorder.

A second report gives a different result, finding an increase in the volume of the amygdala but not the hippocampus [177]. The control group received prolonged exposure and showed a similar decrease in symptoms to the eye movement group, but no increase in brain volume. This evidence suggests that eye movement desensitization causes an increase in the number of neurons.

10.8 INCLUDING INTEROCEPTION

We have to note the importance of interoception. Recall from Chapter 3 that emotions are constructions, or inferences, based on body sensations. Examples of other body sensations are warm, cold, different kinds of pain and itchiness, another person's touch, muscle positions, stretch, cardiac signals, bladder urgency, colonic pressure, hunger, thirst, nausea, and our male and female sexual feelings respectively. The collective noun for these body signals is interoception and the resulting generic emotional label is affect. A bad affect indicates difficulties, such as bodily problems or a future need for food or energy.

These body signals are received in the insular cortex, a brain structure in the middle of the brain, to put that simply for our purposes here [178]. The insular cortex has a topographical map of the various signals for the various body senses. This is in the same sense that the visual cortex has a topographical map of the visual field. When we ask our patients to imagine the distress images, we are activating the image in the visual cortex, and no doubt other places. Similarly, we can claim that the physical sensations that correlate with the distress image, or that might be required to be dealt with as a separate eye movement target, must form a physical sensation image or model in the insular cortex. If we are speculating that artificial PGO signals work in the visual cortex, then we would also want them to influence the insular cortex.

10.9 WORKING CONCLUSIONS ON MOVING EYES

It will not have escaped the reader's attention that much of the above chapter visits many parts of the brain anatomy. In the end, every part is connected to every other part and signals must be transmitted through every location. More than one thing must be happening. There must be a signal of a moving image in the optic nerve and also a proprioceptive signal in the four motor nerves. There must also be a top-down signal to move the eyes, derived from the instructions from the eye movement therapist. Also, the physiological observations show that changes must be occurring throughout the brain. All must be relevant, in some way.

Does our artificial eye movement signal cause events in the brainstem, and more particularly in the pons, that mimic ponto-geniculo-occipital spike trains? We do not know. We do not have any grounds – that I have discovered – to be sure of this, other than that it fits some of the facts. To investigate this, we need a Parkinson's or epilepsy patient with electrodes in the deep brain who needs eye movement therapy. This is not going to happen soon, because eye movement therapy would be contraindicated in such cases. However, we do know that auditory signals can cause ponto-geniculo-occipital spikes when the subject is awake, which gives us a point of contact with the auditory version of eye movement therapy.

Can we attribute a desensitization function to ponto-geniculo-occipital spike trains? The original reason that inspired this was that they were associated with dreams and dreams indicated at least consolidation, if not desensitization. This idea is challenged by the material above but remains a helpful theory if we are looking for a way of implementing the model of reverse learning in the real brain (which we are). Reverse learning also gives us a bridge to working memory accounts of eye movement desensitization. Therefore, I suggest we preserve the ponto-geniculo-occipital spikes, rapid eye movement and reverse learning route to understanding eye movement desensitization.

Perhaps we can assert that artificial eye movements might enable us to control some mechanism that normally, or mostly, acts during rapid eye movement sleep without needing to constrain that mechanism to rapid eye movement sleep. The mechanism can be co-opted in the absence of rapid eye movement sleep. We do not have to say that any particular mechanism or function that we are interested in is the reason for rapid eye movement sleep, as discussed in the next chapter.

Note that slow eye movements also occur during dreaming and sleep cognition because they are happening all the sleep time. If we associate dreaming with rapid eye movement sleep because they happen at the same time, then this is equal grounds for associating dreaming with slow eye movements. Our method of explanation here is to speculate that artificial eye movements inspire some neural pulse in the brain, which might look like something required by reverse learning theory. This requires a brain site for the neural pulse, whether natural or artificial. One premise of this attempt at explanation is that it is the same location in the brain. Perhaps this premise is suspect. There are three possible reasons for this.

The first reason may be that the recovery function of brain neurons may not require allocation to any particular part of the brain. Patients with a stroke or other brain damage can still sleep. Therefore, the whole brain, or any particular part of it, or any sleep stage associated with any part of it, is not required for sleep. It may be that parts of the brain sleep when the brain's owner is awake. Sleep may occur in any brain region, or set of neurons, that has been used up to some limit where recovery is needed.

The physiology of sleep can be reduced further. In-vitro cultures of brain cells show sleep-like states [179]. Cortical neurons from rats were separated and allowed to grow into a network in vitro on an array of micro-electrodes that could pick up any signal. This culture developed a waveform signal at 1 to 3 Hz. This resembles the delta wave frequency of non-rapid eye movement sleep (N 3). Perhaps artificial eye movements may hijack a mechanism that exists in all brain cells, not any particular bit of the brain.

The second reason our method of explanation can be challenged is that it is locationist. This means we are trying to assign specific functions to specific brain locations, based on a premise that locating the function makes for an explanation. This may not work well. Brain imaging methods attempt to locate what we can call here 'mental faculties' at locations in the brain specific for that faculty. Mental faculties might be images, emotions, cognitions or perceptions. These things we need to assess, as discussed in Chapter 3.

We consider here the emotion fear and its possible location in the amygdala. There are two theories here, the locationist and the constructionist. A locationist theory requires that an emotion category, such as fear, is always associated with increased activity in its own place in the brain or a network of places and nowhere else. The usual candidate for fear is the amygdala. Recall from above that eye movement therapy has been found to enlarge the amygdala.

The constructionist theory of emotion says that emotions emerge from more basic brain events not specific to the emotional labels we construct for them. These basic brain events happen in large-scale networks that interact to produce psychological events. This would be shown by brain imaging that showed the same location switches on for several emotions, such as fear, disgust, anger or happiness. Or perhaps a location switches on for some more abstract event, such as core affect or attention.

Results from brain imaging show that mental faculties defined as we see them from outside the brain are not anatomically or physiologically defined in this way [180]. In locationist theory, the amygdala is the brain place for fear, either by itself or as part of a fear network. There is increased amygdala activity when learning to recognize fear in others, such as when looking at fearful faces. Patients with lesions there do not show the expected fear responses. However, brain scans show that the amygdala is part of a network whose function must be described at a more abstract level. This network decides if external events and sensory information are important for the amygdala's owner. This includes dangerous events that cause fear, but much else besides, such as disgust and sadness. The amygdala is active in orienting responses to stimuli that are important, uncertain, socially relevant or novel, or arousing subjectively or emotionally. One explanation is that the amygdala is active when the brain cannot work out what interoceptive sensations mean, what action is needed or what information is needed from external sources. Uncertainty needs to be reduced and probabilities evaluated. Similarly, the visual cortex, which we wish to implicate in our story, is turned on by visual triggers, but it does more than vision. It is activated by some triggers for fear, anger and disgust.

Therefore, if we cannot locate the fear signal in any fear node in the brain, we cannot reasonably speculate that we can send our desensitization signal through it. We would need to send a signal to the visual cortex, other visual places, other sensory places for other sensory images, the amygdala and the insular cortex, at least. We would need to send signals to the whole brain.

The last reason our method of explanation may not hold is the problem of neural reductionism. This is more speculative and somewhat weird, so I have pushed it up to the next chapter, with all other such matters.

10.10 EXPLAINING TO THE PATIENT

Now we have explained eye movement desensitization to ourselves, we still need an explanation for the patients. We should still describe it as artificial dreaming, despite the caveats and difficulties. I delay the explanation until some success has been achieved and the patient needs to understand why. I usually preface my explanation with the remark that it is common in medical history that a method or a medicine is used when it is known to be safe and effective enough, but before it is explained. A good example is anaesthetics. Every day in our hospital, 80 to 100 patients are put to sleep or into a light coma by pumping gases into their lungs. They wake up after surgery and generally they are fine. Nobody understands how pumping weird gases into the lungs can put people out for a few hours. Eye movement desensitization is in that situation. Having said that, there is a story we can tell that begins to explain it. It is artificial dreaming.

When something bad happens to people, it can cause them problems. They may have flashbacks, or other bad memories, of the event. They often have bad dreams and nightmares. Flashbacks and bad dreams are the same thing, except that one happens during the day and one happens at night. Because of this, they often have sleep problems. Eye movement desensitization is best understood as memory repair by artificial dreaming. When something bad, dangerous or difficult happens, we understand it after dreaming about it. That is the probable reason for dreaming. It is like sorting out a filing cabinet that has become overloaded. If you look at somebody who is dreaming, their eyes are moving from side to side. This is called REM sleep or rapid eye movement sleep.

One explanation of this method is that you can make such memory repair happen artificially. If you are asked to think about a flashback and we move your eyes, it may be that the part of your brain that works when you are dreaming is being switched on from outside. The repair needed might be this. The part of the brain where you do your thinking is called short-term or working memory. Working memory can handle only around seven things at a time, as if it has only seven slots. What each thing is depends on what you are thinking about. Normally this does not trouble us, because information flows through so fast that we do not notice the bottleneck. However, trauma memory or anxiety is caused when our working memory gets blocked up. Depending on how many flashbacks you own and how many things remind you of them, then some of the slots in your working memory will be filled up and blocked. If you have three slots blocked with three flashbacks, then you have only four slots to think with. This is why you have concentration problems and memory problems. The eye movement procedure cleans the flashbacks out of the slots. If you like, it is a form of mental hygiene. When your working memory is clean, then you can think about your current problems, concerns or illness better.

11. END NOTES

This last chapter is a miscellany of issues either left over from the previous chapters or included because I find them interesting, here considered to various degrees as notes. A note is an issue that needs to be noted, but is not developed further here, because this is the last chapter.

11.1 LOOKING BACK THROUGH DEEP TIME

The first leftover issue is the evolutionary biology behind what we are doing. This is not just to pursue my interest in evolutionary biology. Eye movement desensitization gives the impression that we are using some fundamental brain biology and I want to look at that. In a previous chapter, we noted that we are not obliged to explain sleep stages with contemporary functions. The reason for this is one of three interesting stories about the evolutionary context of post-traumatic stress disorder. We will need to distinguish between two concepts: current function and phylogenetic function.

Current function means how that behaviour or organ helps the organism survive and reproduce today. Phylogenetic function means the same thing, but stretched back through deep time. Why did that behaviour or organ evolve in the animal's ancestors? Phylogenetic function is different from current function because the function of a behaviour or organ can change during deep time. One might evolve a limb into a fin to swim but one's descendants might use it to paddle, walk, run, fly or dance. Sleep is discussed below as an example of this.

Post-traumatic stress disorder has not evolved

Post-traumatic stress disorder is a disorder, or illness if you prefer, and is dysfunctional. Therefore, something in the system that produces it is functional, in the sense that it improves survival. This must be the human fear response, which is required to avoid being eaten by predators. In the African Origin, lions, hyenas, raptors and snakes might eat humans and other primates [181]. Bad-tempered beasts, such as elephants and hippopotamuses, should also be avoided. Such risks still exist for many people. Animals that avoid predators for long enough will reproduce and pass on their genes. Escaping by running away is expensive in energy and we need to minimize our energy expenditure. No animal can afford to spend all its time running. Therefore, we need to recover from, or limit, the escape response. Running away from a predator uses the same ability as chasing down prey as the predator. Humans are the only ape to have evolved to run down prey in open country. We have physical features, which distinguish us from chimpanzees, that enable us to run [182]. These include psychological abilities as well as physical ones. The escape response must also be the chase response. Let us add them together and call it the running response.

Since most victims of bad life events get over their misfortune, it is likely that post-traumatic stress disorder and other anxiety and distress disorders are a failure to recover from the running response. Therefore, there must be some recovery mechanism that does not depend on the attention or skills of the more recently evolved psychological therapist. Perhaps procedures such as eye movements exploit this mechanism.

Why sleep and sleep stages?

In deep time, the prototype mammal shared a common ancestor with the prototype reptile. This ancestor is the ancestral amniote. 'Amniote' is the collective noun for reptiles, birds, mammals and their precursors, defined by the ability to reproduce with an egg that can survive on land. Reptiles are poikilothermic (or cold-blooded), which means they need the sun to keep warm. Therefore, reptiles are less likely to be nocturnal. At night, reptiles will stop moving and rest, but this state differs physiologically from mammalian sleep. A reptile will become active at dawn and find a sunny place to bask until it warms up. Next on the job list is a period of risk assessment. This calls for a safe place, head dipping, eye movements and body stretching. Having done that, it moves on to the business of the day in short bursts of activity. These alternate with stop periods, during which it scans its environment for risks through orientation reflexes, alarm calls and freezing responses. The ancestral amniote probably had a similar daytime agenda to contemporary reptiles.

The first mammals are descended from this ancestral amniote. However, mammals are homeothermic (or warm-blooded), meaning they can maintain their body temperature independently of the environment. The original reason, or reasons, for homeothermy is not known but must be persuasive, since warming blood uses ten times more oxygen than not warming it. One reason may be passive immunity against fungal infections, since most fungi cannot grow over 37°C [183]. Having achieved homeothermy, you no longer need the sun to warm up. You can become nocturnal, being active at night and sleeping during the day. This is safer, because you can hide in your burrow in the daylight to avoid being eaten by the dinosaurs. Therefore, the daytime behavioural stages of basking and risk assessment would have gone underground. In the millions of years that mammals spent hiding in holes in the ground, perhaps the amniote's daytime behaviour evolved into daytime mammal sleep phases [184,185].

When the dinosaurs became extinct, the mammals came out of their burrows and into the daylight. (Or about half did; the rest are still nocturnal.) Those that did became diurnal – that is, active in the day and resting at night. When they moved to night rest, they were then obliged to keep the same brain behaviour stages. After millions of years in a hole in the ground, these stages had become more fixed and hard-wired in the brain. We now call these stages 'sleep'. The daytime sleep stages became night-time sleep stages. Non-rapid eye movement sleep corresponds to basking and rapid eye movement sleep corresponds to risk assessment. Therefore, any offline fear processing function of mammalian rapid eye movement sleep may originate in the awake threat detection behaviour of the ancestral amniote.

This is an interesting story that mitigates some of the difficulties with explaining eye movement desensitization by comparison with rapid eye movement sleep. However, objections can be made. It is the logic of palaeontology that there are always older fossils in the rock waiting to be found, so this story may change. This timeline may need some modification because nocturnal adaptations first appear in the synapsid line 100 million years before they became mammals [186]. Synapsids are mammals and pre-mammals, those amniotes that are neither reptiles nor birds. There were also nocturnal dinosaurs [187]. However, one does not need to be a mammal to dislike being eaten, and it is probably easier to dodge small theropods in the dark.

Another difficulty is the diversity of rapid eye movement sleep and other sleep behaviours. All animals have some kind of behaviour that looks like sleep. It often contains rhythmic states. Birds have a rapid eye movement sleep that is similar to mammalian rapid eye movement sleep, but have spent the past 300 million years in the trees, not holes in the ground.

Bird brains are different from mammal brains, so this could be an example of convergent evolution. The final difficulty in using rapid eye movement sleep as an explanatory template is that it has not been explained itself [188].

However, the take-home point is that we can locate the original reason for sleep stages in deep time, perhaps in an epoch of nocturnal existence or some other past contingency. To be clear, the original reason in deep time for rapid eye movement sleep could be a period of vigilance while awake in daytime. This shifted to the night-time as millions of years of deep time passed in a hole in the ground. When we take this idea, we can worry less about allocating any function that we want to use to explain our problem to any sleep stage.

Rapid eye movement sleep has functions, but these are either original functions of a waking vigilance period or perhaps acquired later. Other functions might be loaded onto this period because they have to happen at some time and there are only 24 hours in the day, some of which are dark and cold when the planet is turned away from the sun. Rapid eye movement sleep has things in common with waking [189]. One function attributed to rapid eye movement sleep in humans is to rehearse threats [190]. Other maintenance functions may be allocated to sleep time. For example, more sleep correlates with more white blood cells and fewer infections [191]. Sleep improvement is reported with eye movement desensitization. Perhaps eye movement therapy has improved the immune status of my patients with human immunodeficiency virus.

We can also connect this to sleep paralysis, which we often need to include in eye movement desensitization. This is the change of brain state from non-rapid eye movement sleep to rapid eye movement sleep to awake but without the body catching up. Patients with sleep paralysis report the impression that there is something dangerous in the room. Perhaps this is the predator. If the brain gets stuck in the rapid eye movement stage it is in ancestral predator-detection mode.

Historical note about sleep

There may also have been changes in sleep sequence in historical times. Before our romantic primitive lifestyle was corrupted by electric light and modern work schedules, people did not sleep straight through the night. Sleep was divided into two parts; first sleep and second sleep [192]. First sleep was from nightfall to about midnight. Then people awoke and became active to various degrees. After an hour of two, sleep was resumed until daybreak. Presumably, our sleep stages still occurred, but in a more fragmented pattern. If subjects are taken out of normal lighting then, during short photoperiods, human sleep is biphasic [193].

Visual evolution is predator driven

The human visual system may have evolved to break the camouflage of predatory snakes [194,195]. Primates evolved about 60 million years ago. They were nocturnal arboreal animals that ate fruit and insects. Eating fruit confers two assets. Good colour vision is needed to find ripe fruit, which is a good source of glucose. Primates could then neglect the sense of smell, leaving space in the brain to expand the visual system. The two kinds of predatory snakes are constrictors and venomous snakes. Constrictors appeared about 100 million years ago and no doubt preyed upon early mammals. Poisonous snakes appeared at about the same time as the first primates, when primates would have been small enough to eat. Most contemporary primates are too large to be eaten by poisonous snakes, but can still be killed by an attack from a snake defending itself or in a bad temper. Primates in Africa and Asia have been at risk from poisonous snakes for their whole evolutionary careers. African and Asian monkeys and apes have trichromatic visual systems that are closely associated with the fear networks of the brain. They also show innate snake fear.

Physiological investigation of visual cells shows the highest responses to patterns such as moving lines, contrasting dots or diamond patterns that resemble snake skin patterns. Therefore, our ability to see depth, colour and pattern, and to perceive and rotate images, may be founded in the detection of threat. Images communicating fear and distress are our inheritance.

11.2 TWO PROBLEMS IN EVALUATING EYE MOVEMENT DESENSITIZATION

I dropped a chapter that attempted to review evaluations and trials from an earlier version of this work. This was for reasons of space, but it must be said that randomized controlled trials are difficult to summarize. For a 30-year review of trials, see de Jongh et al [196]. However, I want to note two issues. The first issue follows from the theory and practice of eye movement therapy as advocated in this book. In a trial, all distress images to all reported distress triggers should be treated. I predict an average of seven, plus or minus two, or tending in that direction.

I find the second issue rather odd. The randomized controlled trial requires two groups called 'control' and 'experimental'. They are treated the same, except that the experimental group get the new treatment or medicine. They are compared to the control group, who receive treatment as usual. In our case, that is usually some cognitive behaviour method that requires the patient to do homework. Homework might be revisiting a bad life event location, if practical and safe, or listening to their own recorded account repeatedly. The patients receiving eye movement therapy are not asked to do homework because that is not needed. Therefore, in a head-to-head trial, the cognitive behaviour patients are getting more therapy time than the eye movement patients.

Some trials seem to ignore this, while some take it into account. Here is a randomized controlled trial that measured this treatment time difference [197]. Twenty patients with post-traumatic stress disorder were allocated eye movement desensitization or prolonged exposure treatment groups. Each received twelve 90-minute sessions of therapy over 6 weeks. Patients were reassessed after treatment and at 3 and 6 months post treatment. Both treatments reduced symptoms. Treatment time was defined as the total hours exposed to the trauma memories. either in session or as homework. Eye movement desensitization patients needed 21 hours on average, compared with 63 hours for prolonged exposure. Eye movement desensitization reduced more distress in the first appointment. Eye movement desensitization revealed and treated 4.2 trauma memories on average, compared with 1.5 for prolonged exposure. I will not pursue further references here, but please keep this in mind next time you read a trial report.

11.3 TREATING CHRONIC PAIN PATIENTS

Experience in the pain clinic convinced me of the necessity of developing eye movement desensitization with chronic pain patients. This was earlier featured in Chapter 7 as a possible different target, but I wish to emphasize the issue. There are three ways our method can help pain patients.

The first is that it will improve sleep. Second, it will clean up working memory. Many pain patients will report issues on their bad life events list other than pain and disease. Child abuse victims turn up in pain clinics like everywhere else. They may have flashbacks to the accident or misfortune that qualified them for the pain. They may have flashbacks to the worst, or most embarrassing, episodes of pain, other medical misadventures, medical treatment, family members in similar difficulties or dying. They may have flashforwards to a worse situation, which might be a reasonable fear or unreasonable anxiety. This might be called catastrophizing, a common assessment needed by pain patients. More catastrophizing means more pain, or at least more pain-related disability [198]. Eye movement desensitization should first be aimed at these images. There may be improvements in pain. Back pain caused by an accident may change favourably, but complex regional pain syndrome will not. However, the complex regional pain patient might be pleased to be rid of child abuse flashbacks. Even if this does not reduce the pain intensity, it might improve their ability to cope with the pain. They may have nausea or other physical sensations associated with their pain, to which treatment can be directed. If this gives an improvement, it may be worth aiming eye movements at the pain.

Third, eye movement desensitization can work if the experienced pain forms pain images. The premise here is that pain can cause pain images in memory, in the same way that vision forms visual images. Perhaps the difference between pain images and visual images is that the external visual stimulus goes away but the chronic pain stimulus may stay present if due to damaged pain nerves or other injury. Pain images are interoception – that is, an internal sensation for the body. The pain signal will arrive in a topographical pattern in the insular cortex. Perhaps pain that decreases with eye movements is pain image and pain that does not is a continuing pain signal arriving from the body.

Some pain clearly does behave like an image. A woman patient being desensitized to a flashback of a miscarriage reported the same abdominal pain returning. The focus was switched to just the pain, which decreased to zero. She was no longer pregnant or miscarrying, so the pain must have been an image. I recommend that eye movement desensitization in the pain clinic is first directed at any flashbacks detected, to any other report of distress images, then any flashforwards, then any pain images or sensations. Clean up the working memory first, then see what can be done with the pain. Is the pain an image or a signal? If it is an image, it will go away. If it is a signal, does it help if all the other rubbish is cleared out of the topographically organized working memory space in the insular cortex?

Pain patients report imagery [199]. A rescripting method of treating pain images showed good results for pain and anxiety [200]. Rescripting is cognitive therapy to revise catastrophizing thoughts linked to an image. There is evidence that eye movement desensitization can be helpful for pain [201]. However, we should enquire what the eye movements are aimed at in such reports. For example, supplementing other methods of controlling migraine headaches with eye movements increases their effectiveness. However, these eye movements were not being directed at distressing imagery and the patients were not assessed for that [202]. A trial in which back pain patients received eye movement desensitization for past issues followed by treatment for pain flashbacks, flashforwards and sensations had a good effect, including a reduction in pain intensity and disability [203]. We must hope that further research and development of eye movement therapy will be supported and reported from pain clinics. The arguments here probably also apply to other medical, or medically unexplained, symptoms.

11.4 THE BRAIN MAY NOT BE THE WHOLE STORY

I was reminded, in researching for Chapter 10, of the problem of neural determinism. Effectively I am using the word 'determinism' here in a similar away to 'locationist' in the previous chapter, but with extra emphasis. It may not be possible to determine, locate or reduce psychological or cognitive functions to some mechanism occurring at a brain location [204]. Neural determinism is the idea that it is possible and useful to locate psychological function X in brain part Y. Certainly, if function X disappears if there is a lesion at Y, then location Y is originating, or at least channelling, it.

However, pursuing neural determinism reaches a roadblock. It is sometimes observed that as the Y lesion gets larger, functions do not drop out as we might expect. Cases are known in which a patient's normal cognitive function is preserved, more or less, in the absence of large parts of their brain tissue, including up to half of the cortex. When brain scanning was invented, a series of adults who had been treated as children for hydrocephalus were followed up and scanned [205]. The brain ventricles of a child with hydrocephalus are blocked for some reason, such as spina bifida. The pressure of the cerebral spinal fluid increases until the brain tissue is squashed against the skull. In 10% of adults who were followed up, the surgical implantation of a shunt (a tube to drain the fluid down into the body) had not repaired this pathology. This had left a large proportion of the cranium still filled with fluid. The follow-up showed that half of these adults had normal intelligence.

Similar results have been found for children who have had a hemispherectomy for hemiplegia or epilepsy. This operation removes all or most of one half of the cortex, in patients whose condition is so serious that this surgery is worth the risk. When these patients are followed up, the usual result is that there is little or no loss in intelligence scores, and sometimes an improvement. Of course, these children were cognitively disadvantaged to start with, but it is notable that there is so little change after losing half the cortex [206, 207].

It is possible to say that brain development is flexible and such children develop cognitive abilities back into the good half of the cortex. However, this is rather a lot of neurons to lose. There is also the difficulty of explaining how the brain knows how to do this when so much of it is lost. There are also adult cases who complain of some motor difficulty and are brain scanned, and it is discovered that much of their brain tissue is missing. Another observation is that certain animals for example, birds such as crows and rooks, or octopuses, which are not even vertebrates can do interesting tricks such as tool use. These are animals of very little brain, so how do they do this? It becomes increasingly difficult to understand how brains apparently so small or different can carry so much information or perform such tasks.

The explanation attempted in Chapter 10 originally reached for the neural deterministic explanation, but ended by needing to implicate the whole brain. It is necessary to achieve a physiological understanding of eye movement desensitization, but this roadblock may be ahead. Note that it is the psychological working memory explanation that contributes best to the advice given above, not the attempt at physiology.

11.5 ANALOGUE NEURONS AND HOLOGRAPHIC IMAGES

The message from the last note is how little we know about the working of neurons and brains. It is accepted that each neuron fires a nerve impulse, or spike, and that information is coded in some way in the timing between the spikes. This is a frequency-modulated code. We can imagine the brain working in vast networks of such neurons. We considered the function of trains of spikes, ponto-geniculo-occipital trains, as a candidate in explaining eye movement desensitization. Do we mimic this when we move the patient's eyes?

What if this is wrong? While researching this chapter, I found the web book *Rewiring Neuroscience*, which explores a different idea [208]. This starts from the observation that certain animal behaviours happen too fast to be accounted for by the action of a frequency-modulated code in the neurons, as conventionally described. A flying bat can avoid an obstacle too fast for conventional requency-modulatedneurons to signal that need. This leads to a theory that each neuron has lots of channels, say 300, arranged in a helix round the nerve cell body. Each channel has a different value, which increases logarithmically round the helix of 300 channels, so each has a distinct identity. This analogue system transmits signals directly, as analogue images, without the need for a digital code, within a visually organised brain that stores images in a way that is holographic rather than connectionist. As I understand it, this has interesting implications for eye movement desensitization. This book is speculative, but you might like to try it.

11.6 IMPLICIT THEORIES OF THE MIND

We considered neural determinism above and found we can entertain doubts about it. Determinism is the position that one cause is sufficient to explain our problem, or at least that other causes can be deprecated. This is often implicit rather than stated. There is nothing intrinsically wrong with determinism. This book is based on image determinism. However, using the word 'determinism' gives us a handle to identify and dispute certain assumptions. For example, we can identify that many rhetorical methods and models of psychotherapeutic change are rhetorical determinism. By identifying this, I can assert that it does not mean that it can trump my advocacy of image determinism.

In my experience of discussion and advocacy of eye movement desensitization, the conversation can take an odd turn. It is as if one loses some implicit script with the person one is addressing. On these occasions, perhaps I have parted company with that person's implicit model or theory of mind or behaviour. Their theory of mind is cognitively, or at least linguistically, determined. Perhaps listening to your own self-talk can lead to the assumption that another's self-talk determines the other's mind or behaviour.

We cannot assume that completing the narrative cures the patient or alleviates their life issues, or whatever expression one uses for improving the patient. Psychological therapy is not about completing, or explaining, the life history of the patient. I am not saying that a patient should not understand their life. We should all live an examined life and we all prefer to think that our life is based on a true story. We would all like our lives to be explained. However, I argue that there is no logical necessity to claim that is the job of a psychological therapist.

11.7 EMOTIONAL DETERMINISM

We can also consider emotional determinism here. I found this idea in Furedi's necessary book *Therapy Culture* [209]. Emotional determinism is the belief that emotions are the primary cause of behaviour or states of mind. An emotion is the origin of our actions. A statement of emotions trumps any more logical enquiry after the facts or a more considered judgement. An implicit premise of emotional determinism may prevent acceptance that the patient can be helped by systematic eye movements directed at toxic images, in which questioning about emotions is regarded as secondary to measuring with numbers.

We should note another issue with emotional determinism. There is risk of a rhetorical trap because questioning an emotional statement can be construed as offensive. Since an accusation of offensiveness is another emotional statement, challenging it may attract a further charge of offensiveness.

No evidence may be offered to support this charge because any defence offered may also be considered offensive. More generally, we can notice this is a common rhetorical device. Alice accuses Bob of some error such that the error, or it's context, has some property such that if Bob defends himself, the error is compounded into a sin. Result: Bob apologises and falls silent. This should have a Latin tag, but I have not been able to find one. We could call it the ad hominem booby trap.

We need to be aware of these issues caused by implicit emotional determinism. If emotions are the labels put on interoceptive signals and depend on an experiential, linguistic or social convention, then we are allowed to question such conventions. We can do this without being considered impolite or offensive. We can interview and treat our patients in the straightforward manner advocated in this book. We can allow that the degree of emotional harm, or strain, from the stress of a bad life event can vary. When we do this, we are not being disrespectful or careless of our patient's rights or needs.

11.8 THE EFFECTS OF CHILD SEXUAL ABUSE CAN VARY

We briefly visit the problems of child sexual abuse in particular. The argument also addresses other forms of child abuse. I do so with some caution, because in some people's eyes, anything considered less than unconditional condemnation may be considered exculpation of child abuse. Exculpating child abusers is not what I am discussing here. The issue is that helping their victims needs a clear head and one of the things we need to be clear about is that the bad effects of child sexual abuse can vary. The effects can vary across time in one person or between people [210].

I recommend that psychological distress, legal culpability and moral outrage be considered as separate categories. This separation must be made clearly for sexual abuse and assault. The difficulty here is that sexual assault, especially child sexual abuse, inspires disgust and sympathy. The appeal to disgust is powerful, but should be recognized and not trump a more logical or factual approach. Disgust, and the related emotion of moral outrage, should not determine our clinical responses or opinions.

This disgust can cause the assumption that psychological harm always results. In fact, psychological harm from child abuse can vary, in a similar way to that from other bad life events. We must again distinguish between stress and strain. The stress event may be serious, disgusting, illegal and morally reprehensible, but the resulting strain may be less. Disgust does not permit us to assume strain equals stress. Moral outrage and disgust do not validate or require psychological harm. Moral outrage and disgust do not mean the victim cannot be helped. Moral outrage and disgust do not mean that victims need to suffer all their lives, or in some way remain a symbol of that outrage. Moral outrage and disgust do not prove the guilt of those accused of committing the offence, as seems to be sometimes assumed. They are innocent until proven guilty, which is a legal decision that depends on evidence and the decision of a court.

There is a related issue with child sexual abuse. When it happens, the child may not experience it as bad. The child may think this is normal play or affection. Only later, with the advent of adult understanding, does it become distressing. Possibly it may not become distressing even at that time, even if understood to be a moral outrage or an unwise, immature life choice. We can determine distress by the distress score, not our feeling of moral outrage on hearing the story. This may require a discussion with the patient ('It must have been my fault it happened, because I did not stop it').

11.9 TAXONOMY OF PATIENTS

Here is an informal taxonomy of the various kinds of patients who should or should not receive eye movement treatment.

1. The usual suspects

The most common type of patient will report distressing images to bad life events. Examples are rape, child abuse, domestic abuse, assault, combat or accidents. They can also be medical incidents, such as the worst episodes of pain, receiving a diagnosis, medical accidents, childbirth trauma or other illness. The bad memories might be episodic or semantic. An episodic memory is a record of one event, labelled with time and place. Eye movement treatment with a semantic image will work most of the time, but may decompose into episodes. Patients will also report distress images to life events that we might not consider distressing. Some people are as distressed by the death of a dog or horse as a human. Our attention to such life events will be guided by the distress, or strain, score given by the patient, not our opinion about what is traumatic. Some patients may report images to future life events or hallucinations. The patient will show distress, which can range from a fleeting expression to a major upset. For a major upset, one asset of eye movement desensitization, as advised here, is that the therapist need assess only the first, and perhaps the second, flashback to decide if the patient is eligible. There is no need to cause further distress by going through all possible flashbacks.

2. Patients with other difficult life events

The indication for eye movement desensitization is the report of distressing images. It is not post-traumatic stress disorder or any particular life event, whether traumatic, toxic or just distressing. A panic patient may just report distressing images to panics without any originating life event. It is also possible to accept a patient for eye movement desensitization who will also need some other method of help. For example, eye movement desensitization may not be helpful for obsessive-compulsive disorder. However, such cases can receive eye movement desensitization if they report distressing imagery. An attempt can be made to treat flashforwards to the house burning down if the oven is not checked an even number of times. This problem usually gives the impression of being more cognitively determined than image determined, so any benefit may reverse.

A patient may require help for one thing, but not another. One man requested help for his child abuse history, but did not need treatment for his job history as an accident investigator, which required dealing with the remains of accident victims.

3. Resilient patients

Patients with good self-control may not show obvious distress, but are still candidates. Some patients stay relaxed, competent and in command of their sense of humour. The indication is identification and measurement of distress images. They might be resilient people or have been carrying their bad memories for a long time. The distress triggers may affect only one part of their life, such as sexual relations or work. In the same way that some people have a high tolerance of physical pain, some people can carry their emotional pain. Probably the same people.

4. Patients with incomplete reports

A candidate may report their history with something apparently missing. There can be various reasons for this, as listed in Chapter 3. This may be an accident victim who sustained concussion. They might have taken alcohol, or some other drug, before the trauma. They might report they were given a drug by somebody else to facilitate rape. The patient may not first report a visual flashback if their vision was obscured during an assault. Memory loss can be the initial presentation of post-traumatic stress disorder, rather than any obvious distress. Such a patient may present through a memory clinic rather than psychiatric or medical referral.

On occasion, the patient appears unable to report the most difficult part of their history. Some patients will report a feeling as if some distressing memory is blocked in some way. Others are puzzled and need an explanation of possible reasons for the memory gap. The missing episode may include physical contact, such as an assault, injury or painful medical treatment. Such patients may be distressed, but this may not be obviously linked to their story, at least as initially understood. Their distress may increase slowly as the discussion approaches the dangerous area. For example, a road traffic accident victim may not have a flashback to the accident itself, but become distressed about some other aspect of the event. Examples are imagining explaining to their colleagues why they were off work or being visited while in hospital. Treatment should start on these targets and the patient may remember the rest. However, a life event not previously reported can be remembered without any warning signs.

Why does this happen? It might simply be a new report from the patient. The interview recommended for the first appointment avoids asking for all details about all bad life events. The briefing warns patients that they may remember something painful. As discussed elsewhere, we are not going to call this repression, dissociation or anything dramatic because we do not need to. Chapter 3, on remembering, gives reasons for non-reporting. Such distressing memories are the next target for eye movement desensitization. The remedies for high distress are presented in Chapter 8.

5. Patients who do not consent

The patient may not agree to eye movement desensitization when the therapist considers it indicated. Since we can only proceed with patient consent, there is nothing we can do about this. A patient may report that they do not need treatment because they can deal with the problem themselves. Others may feel unworthy of treatment for some reason, such as the self-blame reported by child abuse victims. Such patients may be depressed and believe that no change is possible. A self-sufficient rape victim may take the 'strong woman' act too far and refuse treatment. The therapist should respond that just because they can carry the load does not mean they should. Such patients may have a military background. In which case, the therapist should observe that carrying flashbacks in their rucksack may be necessary during military service but is not required in civilian life. Eye movement desensitization will relieve them of this burden. The long-term consequences of refusing treatment could be depression, bad decision-making or bad relationships.

6. Recovered patients

There are also patients with a memory of events for which distress might be expected but who remain calm and have low distress scores. Such patients usually, but not always, also report fuzzy images rather than clear ones. The patient will be able to control the images ('I just think of something else'). These patients have experienced bad life events but have never suffered from distress memories, or have recovered without help, or with other previous help. There might be a partial recovery.

The bad life events that could be anticipated to be toxic, such as rape, may have low distress scores because of the passage of time, but the social phobia and sleep paralysis might still need attention. However, before concluding this, the therapist should determine if the patient belongs in one of the above categories. Natural recovery is common, but cannot be assumed in people who arrive at the clinic.

7. Some patients are beyond any help

The author once met a patient with a 60-year history of child abuse, difficult war experiences, an abusive marriage of 50 years and chronic pain. The author was naïve enough to explain eye movement desensitization to her. She refused on the grounds that it was too late. There are people who have suffered in ways that may have profound medical, military, moral, personal, legal or political implications for them. I recommend that you try to help them, but be prepared to recognize this and say that to them.

11.10 SOME PATIENT REPORTS ARE NOT TRUE

Sometimes the patient's story develops lacunae. Here are two examples. In both of these cases some doubt could be construed in the story, but not sufficient to stop treatment.

1. A patient reported a sexual assault that allegedly occurred under circumstances unusually dishonourable for even such an event. The eye movement desensitization proceeded without causing sufficient suspicion to suspend the treatment. It was later evident that there was no assault.
2. A military veteran reported that he had participated in a military action that resulted in a serious war crime. Eye

movement desensitization reduced distress images, none of which concerned the alleged event. He dropped out of treatment. A later web search found two reports of this action, both of which made it clear the alleged crime did not happen.

An extraordinary report was published in 2005 [211]. It concerned 100 American men enrolled in a Veteran's Administration treatment program for veterans of the Vietnam war. They had requested treatment for combat post-traumatic stress disorder and depression. All these patients were diagnosed using validated questionnaires. Using the United States Freedom of Information Act, the researchers requested the military record of each patient. Of the 100 help-seeking patients, it was discovered that 42 had served in Vietnam and had documented evidence of combat exposure. Twenty had been in Vietnam, but with an unclear combat record. Another 32 had been in Vietnam, but had no combat record. Of the rest, two had been in the military but it was not recorded if they had ever served in Vietnam, two were in the military but had not served in Vietnam, and the last two had never been in the military at all. Those patients who were proven non-combatants were reporting combat flashbacks. This symptom of over-reporting or falsification is sufficiently characteristic of military patients that it is a research subject by itself.

A particular subset of the reporting problem concerns rape and sexual assaults. My interest in this subject was sharpened when first drafting this chapter because at the same time I was dealing with four (probable or proven) fake rape presentations.

This includes the case summarized above. This was in a sexual health clinic, which sees genuine rape victims. How many rape allegations are not true? This is a dangerous area, since writing a sceptical opinion risks an imputation of lack of concern for victims. However, we must note the problem exists and diverts resources from genuine victims. There is some research. The review chapter of the *Rape Investigation Handbook* cites eight research papers giving false reporting rates of between 8% and 41% [212]. This is a difficult area and much can happen between an alleged assault and the conviction of an assailant that we will not consider here. However, the message here is that some patients do not tell the truth and this may impact their eye movement treatment.

We should not assume that patients whose reports are not veridical or true are lying with intent to deceive. There are five possible realities for a report of a bad life event:

1. It is true.
2. It is not true but for some reason, the patient believes it to be true. This is tolerable. It may be caused by memory failings, as discussed elsewhere. It may be a part of the depression or a symptom of the distress illness.
3. It is not true but something else about the case is. It is possible to doubt part of the report when another part is proven.
4. It is not true. The patient knows it is not true and is lying with the intent to deceive. This is an issue for the patient, who has broken the moral contract implicit between healer and patient.
5. We should remember that reports that lose touch with reality may be delusional and part of a psychotic illness.

We cannot prove that a patient is insincere. There will never be a method or machine that can demonstrate or prove dishonesty, because that would require proof that the index event had not happened. By my understanding of logic, it is impossible to prove a negative proposition. However, these three signs might cause suspicion:

1. Over time, the story becomes more elaborate, more horrible and less convincing. The report fails to achieve consilience. Imagine a jigsaw puzzle where the pieces fail to fit.
2. The patient shows low or strange emotional or physiological reactivity, despite reporting a high distress score.
3. The patient does not improve with treatment.
4. The patient fails to comply and avoids eye contact.

A patient may show each of these signs for valid reasons, considered as problems elsewhere. When these signs combine over time and cannot be solved, then suspicions should be aroused. A patient may show none of these signs and still be insincere. The reporting of symptoms by patients is subjective, so it is not possible to distinguish between genuine subjective symptoms reported sincerely and less sincere reports. What can we do about this problem? I am not sure, but here are some notes:

1. Some people can be allowed to lie because previously they needed to lie to avoid abuse, injury or death.
2. Instead of thinking that the report is either true or false, consider a truth scale from 0% to 100%. All patients begin with 100% prior credibility and then lose or regain credibility with more experience and information.

3. Consider whether an answer needs to be 100% credible to decide what to do next. The decision to offer eye movement desensitization does not require 100% credibility.
4. One practical advantage of eye movement desensitization is that an image does not have to be veridical. Flashforwards are not veridical.
5. Such patients have been laconically described as time-wasters. Sometimes it might be best to finish such an unproductive appointment as soon as possible, in the interests of the next patient.
6. There is not much that can be done about this problem. We cannot accuse a patient of lying without evidence. Since we are not detectives, it is unlikely we will obtain that evidence. Even if we had it, we could not do anything with it. Challenging a non-patient about a non-illness leads to the patient's departure. We might then miss the real issue the patient is presenting, if that is what is happening.
7. Sometimes we can be sure that the patient is not telling the truth. Some things are physiologically impossible. I also do not believe that my local police force assassinates its prisoners.
8. A false presentation is sometimes called a factitious illness. It is difficult to know what to do with such patients [213].

11.11 CONTRAINDICATIONS

A web search will show various lists of contraindications for eye movement desensitization. This is my list, based on experience, opinion and discussion:

1. Any untreated brain disease. Epilepsy is the obvious example, although there are no doubt others. Epilepsy that is stable on medication, or which has not appeared for a year or more, is acceptable. Some patients report having episodes that may be epilepsy, or are under investigation, or which have been attributed to stress, perhaps correctly. Eye movement desensitization can be indicated in these cases.

2. Any active medical illness causing continuing pain or distress may preclude eye movement desensitization until the situation is resolved. However, it may be that the medical situation could be improved, or treatment facilitated, with successful eye movement desensitization. Imminent surgery precludes eye movement treatment.

3. Uncontrolled alcohol or illegal drug use. There is a dilemma here because the chemical use might be to self-medicate the flashbacks. Perhaps treating the flashbacks will reduce chemical use. However, there is clearly a dangerous level of use that stops treatment.

4. Undiagnosed eye pain stops treatment until it is understood, or indicates the auditory method.

Not contraindications

These should not stop eye movement desensitization treatment:

1. Dissociation can be found on some contraindication lists, but not here. For our purposes now, this may mean two things. If it means severe distress, then it should be managed as part of continuing eye movement therapy. Methods for this are discussed elsewhere. If it means some kind of anomalous presentation, then stop until the situation is evaluated.

2. Pregnancy. I recollect that this was considered a contraindication in the early days of eye movement therapy. I am not clear of the reason for this. I have found myself treating patients who later discovered that they were pregnant. I do not think it is a problem in the first or second trimester, especially if the issue is pregnancy-related. Examples might be a medical phobia preventing antenatal care or sexual abuse history preventing obstetric examinations. Later in the pregnancy, attempts to help might be ill-advised, but by then the woman is more concerned with the new baby. Advise her to return when the infant has arrived and she is able to do that.

3. A very severe and extended trauma history, such as a long history of child or marital abuse, or torture in political refugees. Also, severe distress when discussing trauma history or during treatment. Such cases are often described as complex and therefore unsuitable for eye movement therapy. I disagree and advocate that these are the cases

that our method was invented for. Patients who show high distress when reporting life events are good cases because they are clearly focused on the toxic images. This indicates that eye movement desensitization will relieve that distress.

4. Lack of valid trauma events. The criterion for eye movement treatment is distressing imagery. It does not have to have been caused by actual events. A panic patient may report images of panic attacks, which can be treated, but no originating event.

5. A terminal illness does not preclude eye movement desensitization.

6. Visual disability might be an obvious contraindication. However, this is when the auditory method can be used.

7. Psychotic patients. This is another issue that, like pregnancy, has ascended into the permitted list. It was considered in Chapter 7.

11.12 CHECKLIST

Checklists are often used in healthcare to maintain standards. This is mine.

1. Always check for flashforwards or other images not in the past.

2. If the desensitization slows down or stops, ask for physical sensation and location, which has not yet qualified for a cognitive or emotional label.

3. Always check for vaginal or anal pain in rape victims who get stuck. Not nice, but necessary.

4. Always check for social anxiety in rape victims or patients in their teens and twenties.
5. Always watch out for for sleep problems, of which sleep paralysis is the most important. Other sleep disturbance, such as nightmares and night panics, may be reported.
6. Caution is needed when reporting treatment results. The referrer may know the patient's history. If not, the referrer does not need to know the details, especially of sexual matters. The patient will not want such descriptions on their file for the rest of their life.

11.13 COVID-19

The author is editing this chapter in the lockdown of 2020, and does not have any direct experience of Covid-19 patients. However, a last note on this problem seems a good idea, so here are some suggestions. As you would expect, people exposed to such viruses report depression and anxiety [214]. Survivors of Covid-19 will be at risk of flashbacks to delirium, intensive care experiences and hallucinations. These patients can also experience the sensation of liquid in the lungs, which could be a panic trigger. Colleagues who were assigned to Red Covid-19 wards may return requiring treatment because the death of a patient triggers their own distress memories.

I have no doubt that this infection is a stress but strain is less than stress. Response to the stress can vary between between zero and ten. There will also be recovery over time. Record all bad life events, not just to the the Covid-19 infection and treatment. As with all other illness, disorders and distress triggers, eye movement treatment must be directed at all reported targets, to clear the whole working memory.

REFERENCES & NOTES

[1] American Psychiatric Association (2013) *Diagnostic and Statistical Manual of Mental Disorders* (5th ed.). Washington, DC. Usually known as DSM5.

[2] World Health Organization. *International Statistical Classification of Diseases and Related Health Problems, 10th revision.* Usually known as ICD-10 http://apps.who.int/classifications/apps/icd/icd10online/
Last checked December 2020.

[3] Bradford, H. (1977) *A Short Textbook of Medical Statistics.* Hodder & Stoughton, London. Chapter 24.
This is a classic statement of criteria for illness causality. It cites a number of guidelines for judging causality. I consider only the two relevant to my discussion.

[4] Frissa, S., Hatch, S.L., Gazard, B., Fear, N.T., & Hotopf, M. (2013) Trauma and Current Symptoms of PTSD in a South East London Community. *Social Psychiatry & Psychiatric Epidemiology, 48(8).* 1199–1209.

[5] Jonas, S., Bebbington, P., McManus, S., Meltzer, H., Jenkins, R., Kuipers, EC. Cooper, M., & King Brugha, T. (2011). Sexual Abuse and Psychiatric Disorder in England: results from the 2007 Adult Psychiatric Morbidity Survey. *Psychological Medicine, 41(4).* 709–719.

[6] Logue, M.W., van Rooij, S.J., Dennis, E.L., Davis, S.L., Hayes, JP., Stevens, J.S., et al. (2018) Smaller Hippocampal Volume in Post-traumatic Stress Disorder: a Multisite ENIGMA-PGC Study: Subcortical Volume-try Results from Post-traumatic Stress Disorder Consortia. *Biological Psychiatry, 83 (3).* 244–253.

[7] Gilbertson, M.W., Shenton, M.E., Ciszewski, A., Kasai, K., Lasko, N.B., Orr, S.P., & Pitman, R.K. (2002) Smaller Hippocampal Volume Predicts Pathologic Vulnerability to Psychological Trauma. *Nature Neuroscience, 5 (11).* 1242–1247. https://doi.org/10.1038/nn958

[8] Bodkin, J.A., Pope, H.G., Det ke, M.J., & Hudson, J.I. (2007). Is PTSD Caused by Traumatic Stress? *Journal of Anxiety Disorders, 21 (2).* 176–182.

[9] Franklin, C.L., Raines, A.M., & Hurlocker, M.C. (2019) No Trauma, No Problem: Symptoms of Post-traumatic Stress in the Absence of a Criterion A Stressor. *Journal of Psychopathology & Behavioral Assessment, 41 (1)*. 107–111.

[10] Brewin, C.R., Lanius, R.A., Novac, A., Schnyder, U., & Galea, S. (2009) Reformulating PTSD for DSM-5: Life after Criterion A. *Journal of Traumatic Stress, 22 (5)*. 366–373.

[11] Kilpatrick, D.G., Resnick, H.S., & Acierno, R. (2009) Should PTSD Criterion A be Retained? *Journal of Traumatic Stress, 22 (5)*. 374–383.

[12] Breslau, N., & Alvarado, G.F. (2007) The Clinical Significance Criterion in DSM-IV Post-traumatic Stress Disorder. *Psychological Medicine, 37 (10)*. 1437–1444.

[13] Four books on the background to post-traumatic stress disorder:
    (1.) Young, A. (1995) *The Harmony of Illusions: Inventing Post-Traumatic Stress Disorder*. Princeton University Press.
    (2.) Jones, E. & Wessley, S. (2005) *Shell Shock to PTSD*. Maudsley Monographs, Psychology Press.
    (3.) Rosen, G.M. (2004) *Post-traumatic Stress Disorder; Issues and Controversies*. J. Wiley & Sons.
    (4.) Brewin, C.R. (2003) *Post-traumatic Stress Disorder; Malady or Myth?* Yale University Press.

[14] Rosch, P.J. (2002) *Hans Selye and the Birth of the Stress Concept. A Clinical Guide to the Treatment of the Human Stress Response.* Springer. Chapter 2.

[15] Selye, H. (1978) *The Stress of Life.* McGraw-Hill.
This discussion is in Chapter 3.

[16] Schütte, M. (2009) *Methods for Measuring Mental Stress and Strain. Industrial Engineering and Ergonomics.* Springer. Chapter 30.

[17] Bridger, R.S., Kilminster, S., & Slaven, G. (2007) Occupational Stress and Strain in the Naval Service: 1999 and 2004. *Occupational Medicine, 57 (2).* 92–97.
The questionnaire used to measure strain was the General Health Questionnaire 12, used in psychiatric research to measure anxiety or depression as a result of life events.

[18] Summerfield, D. (2011) Metropolitan Police Blues: Protracted Sickness Absence, Ill Health Retirement, and the Occupational Psychiatrist. *British Medical Journal, 342.* 950–952.

[19] Rutter, M. (1981) Stress, Coping and Development: Some Issues and Some Questions. *Journal of Child Psychology & Psychiatry, 22 (4).* 323–356.

[20] Spector, N.H. (1997) The Great Hans Selye and the Great Stress Muddle. *Developmental Brain Dysfunction, 10 (6).* 538–542.

[21] Kartha, A., Brower, V., Saitz, R., Samet, J.H., Keane, T.M., & Liebschutz, J. (2008) The Impact of Trauma Exposure and Post-traumatic Stress Disorder on Healthcare Utilization Among Primary Care Patients. *Medical Care, 46 (4).* 388–393.

[22] Bloch, S., & Reddaway, P. (1984) *Soviet Psychiatric Abuse.* Victor Gollancz Ltd, London.

[23] Burianova, H., & Grady, C.L. (2007). Common and Unique Neural Activations in Autobiographical, Episodic, and Semantic Retrieval. *Journal of Cognitive Neuroscience, 19 (9).* 1520–1534.

[24] Burton, S., & Blair E. (1991) Task Conditions, Response Formulations and Response Accuracy for Behavioral Frequency Questions in Surveys. *Public Opinion Quarterly,* 55. 50–79.

[25] Schacter, D.L., & Addis, D.R. (2007) The Cognitive Neuroscience of Constructive Memory: Remembering the Past and Imagining the Future. *Philosophical Transactions of the Royal Society B: Biological Sciences, 362 (1481).* 773–786.

[26] Szpunar, K.K., Watson, J.M., & McDermott, K.B. (2007) Neural Substrates of Envisioning the Future. *Proceedings of the National Academy of Sciences, 104 (2).* 642–647.

[27] Schacter D.L. (2000) *The Seven Sins of Memory.* Houghton Mifflin.

[28] I originally wrote *Carry On Cleo* here, but decided that might be an obscure reference for the international readership I aspire to. Research reveals there are 61 films or shows with Cleopatra in the title. (IMDB.com, September 2019.)

[29] Baker R.A. (1992). *Hidden Memories.* Prometheus Books, Buffalo, NY.

[30] Roediger III, H.L. (1996) Memory Illusions. *Journal of Memory & Language, 35 (2).* 76–100.

[31] Howe, M.L. (2013) Memory Development: Implications for Adults [31] Recalling Childhood Experiences in the Courtroom. *Nature Reviews Neuroscience, 14.* 869–876. https://doi.org/10.1038/nrn3627

[32] Wolfer, T.A. (1999). It Happens all the Time: Overcoming the Limits of Memory and Method for Chronic Community Violence Experience. *Journal of Interpersonal Violence, 14 (10).* 1070–1094.

[33] Moffitt, T.E., Caspi, A., Taylor, A., Kokaua, J., Milne, B.J., Polanczyk, G., & Poult on, R. (2010). How Common are Common Mental Disorders? Evidence That Lifetime Prevalence Rates are Doubled by Prospective Versus Retrospective Ascertainment. *Psychological Medicine, 40 (6).* 1–11.
The full list is anxiety, panic, specific phobia, social phobia, generalized anxiety disorder, depression, alcohol dependency

and cocaine dependency. To avoid confusion, this report did not consider trauma events or post-traumatic stress disorder.

[34] Goodman, G.S., Ghetti, S., Quas, J.A., Edelstein, R.S., Alexander, K.W., Redlich, A.D., & Jones, D.P. (2003). A Prospective Study of Memory for Child Sexual Abuse: New Findings Relevant to the Repressed-memory Controversy. *Psychological Science, 14 (2)*. 113–118.

[35] Baldwin, J.R., Reuben, A., Newbury, J.B., & Danese, A. (2019). Agreement Between Prospective and Retrospective Measures of Childhood Maltreatment: a Systematic Review and Meta-analysis. *JAMA Psychiatry*. March 20, 2019. doi:10.1001/jamapsychiatry.2019.0097.

[36] Pope, H.G., Hudson, J.I., Bodkin, J.A., & Oliva, P. (1998) Questionable Validity of Dissociative Amnesia in Trauma Victims. Evidence from Prospective Studies. *The British Journal of Psychiatry, 172 (3)*. 210–215.

[37] McNally, R.J. (2005). *Remembering Trauma*. Harvard University Press.

[38] Bower G.H. (1990) Awareness, The Unconscious and Repression: an Experimental Psychologist's Perspective. *Repression and Dissociation*. University of Chicago.

[39] Rhodes, K.V., Drum, M., Anliker, E., Frankel, R.M., Howes, D.S., & Levinson, W. (2006) Lowering the Threshold

for Discussions of Domestic Violence: a Randomized Controlled Trial of Computer Screening. *Archives of Internal Medicine, 166 (10).* 1107–1114.

[40] Levy, A.G., Scherer, A.M., Zikmund-Fisher, B.J., Larkin, K., Barnes, G.D., & Fagerlin, A. (2018) Prevalence of and Factors Associated With Patient Nondisclosure of Medically Relevant Information to Clinicians. *JAMA Network Open, 1 (7).* e185293-e185293.

[41] Robertson, G. (2010) *The Case of the Pope; Vatican Accountability for Human Rights Abuses.* Penguin.

[42] McNally, R.J., & Geraerts, E. (2009) A New Solution to the Recovered Memory Debate. *Perspectives on Psychological Science, 4 (2).* 126–134.

[43] Luborsky, L., & Barrett, M.S. (2006) The History and Empirical Status of Key Psychoanalytic Concepts. *Annual Review of Clinical Psychology, 2.* 1-19.

[44] Five books on psychoanalysis:
    (1.) Thornton, E.M. (1982) *The Freudian Fallacy: Freud and Cocaine.* Paladin.
    (2.) Eysenck, H. (1985) *Decline and Fall of the Freudian Empire.* Routledge.
    (3.) Crews, F. (1995) *The Memory Wars.* New York Review of Books.
    (4.) Webster, R. (1995) *Why Freud Was Wrong: Sin, Science*

and Psychoanalysis. HarperCollins.

(5) Esterson, A. (1993) *Seductive Mirage: an Exploration of the Work of Sigmund Freud.* Open Court Publishing Co.

[45] Frankel, F.H. (1994) The Concept of Flashbacks in Historical Perspective. *International Journal of Clinical & Experimental Hypnosis, 42 (4).* 321–336.

[46] Deutsch S., & Deutsch A. (1993) *Understanding the Nervous System: An Engineering Perspective.* Wiley.
Listed here are 15 human sensory systems: (1) touch, (2) cold, (3) warmth, (4) pain, (5) auditory (sound), (6) taste, (7) olfactory (smell), (8) visual, (9) blood temperature change, (10) vestibular (balance), (11) chemoreceptor (blood chemistry), (12) baroreceptor (blood pressure), (13) kinaesthetic (angle of joints), (14) spindle (muscle stretch) and (15) force (tendon organs; to limit muscle contraction). All these must contribute to sensory images.

[47] Jacobson, E. (1932) Electrophysiology of Mental Activities. *The American Journal of Psychology, 44 (4).* 677–694.

[48} Antrobus, J.S., & Singer, J.L. (1964) Eye Movements Accompanying Daydreaming, Visual Imagery, and Thought Suppression. *The Journal of Abnormal & Social Psychology, 69 (3).* 244–252.

[49] Singer, J.L., & Antrobus, J.S. (1965) Eye Movements During Fantasies: Imagining and Suppressing Fantasies. *Archives of General Psychiatry, 12 (1).* 71–78.

[50] Deckert, G.H. (1964) Pursuit Eye Movements in the Absence of a Moving Visual Stimulus. *Science, 143.* 1192–1193.

[51] Bensafi, M., Porter, J., Pouliot, S., Mainland, J., Johnson, B., Zelano, C., & Sobel, N. (2003) Olfactomotor Activity During Imagery Mimics That During Perception. *Nature Neuroscience, 6 (11).* 1142–1144.

[52] Decety, J., Jeannerod, M., Germain, M., & Pastene, J. (1991) Vegetative Response During Imagined Movement is Proportional to Mental Effort. *Behavioural Brain Research, 42 (1).* 1–5.

[53] Wandell, B.A., Dumoulin, S.O., & Brewer, A.A. (2007) Visual Field Maps in Human Cortex. *Neuron, 56 (2).* 366–383.

[54] Sartory, G., Cwik, J., Knuppertz, H., Schürholt, B., Lebens, M., Seitz, R.J., & Schulze, R. (2013) In Search of the Trauma Memory: a Meta-analysis of Functional Neuroimaging Studies of Symptom Provocation in Post-traumatic Stress Disorder. *PLOS One, 8 (3).* e58150.

[55] Wolpe, J. (1982) *The Practice of Behavior Therapy.* Pergamon.

[56] Beck, A.T. (1970) Role of Fantasies in Psychotherapy and Psychopathology. *The Journal of Nervous & Mental Disease, 150 (1).* 3–17.

[57] Beck, A.T., & Emery, G. (1985). *Anxiety Disorders and Phobias.* Basic Books.

[58] Ekman, P. (1999) Basic Emotions. *Handbook of Cognition and Emotion.* Wiley. Chapter 3.

[59] Ekman, P.(2003) *Emotions Revealed.* Weidenfeld, London.

[60] Oaten, M., Stevenson, R.J., & Case, T.I. (2009) Disgust as a Disease-Avoidance Mechanism. *Psychological Bulletin, 135 (2).* 303–321.

[61] Curtis, V. (2011) Why Disgust Matters. *Philosophical Transactions of the Royal Society of London. Series B, Biological Sciences, 366 (1583).* 3478–90.

[62] Noakes, T.D. (2012). Fatigue is a Brain-derived Emotion That Regulates the Exercise Behavior to Ensure the Protection of Whole Body Homeostasis. *Frontiers in Physiology, 3, 82.* doi.org/10.3389/fphys.2012.00082

[63] Barrett, L.F. (2017) *How Emotions Are Made: The Secret Life of the Brain.* Pan Macmillan. how-emotions-are-made.com

[64] Stevens, S.S. (1946) On the Theory of Scales of Measurement. *Science, 103.* 677–680.

[65] This is Mohs's scale, relegated to a note since probably not relevant to eye movement treatment: 10, diamond; 9, corundum; 8, topaz; 7, quartz; 6, feldspar; 5, apatite; 4, fluorspar; 3, calcite; 2, gypsum; 1, talc.

[66] Sokolowski, H.M., Fias, W., Ononye, C.B., & Ansari, D. (2017) Are Numbers Grounded in a General Magnitude Processing System? A Functional Neuroimaging Meta-analysis. *Neuropsychologia, 105.* 50–69.

[67] Cantlon, J.F., Platt, M.L., & Brannon, E.M. (2009) Beyond The Number Domain. *Trends in Cognitive Sciences, 13 (2).* 83–91.

[68] Nieder, A., & Dehaene, S. (2009) Representation of Number in the Brain. *Annual Review of Neuroscience, 32.* 185–208.

[69] Harvey, B.M., Klein, B.P., Petridou, N., & Dumoulin, S.O. (2013) Topographic Representation of Numerosity in the Human Parietal Cortex. *Science, 341 (6150).* 1123–1126.

[70] Kutter, E.F., Bostroem, J., Elger, C.E., Mormann, F., & Nieder, A. (2018) Single Neurons in the Human Brain Encode Numbers. *Neuron, 100 (3).* 753–761.

[71] Kim, D., Bae, H., & Park, Y.C. (2008) Validity of the Subjective Units of Disturbance Scale in EMDR. *Journal of EMDR Practice & Research, 2 (1).* 57–62.

[72] Donovan, K.A., Grassi, L., McGinty, H.L., & Jacobsen, P.B. (2014) Validation of the Distress Thermometer Worldwide: State of the Science. *PsychoOncology, 23 (3).* 241–250.

[73] Jacobsen, P.B., Donovan, K.A., Trask, P.C., Fleishman, S.B., Zabora, J., Baker, F., & Holland, J.C. (2005) Screening for Psychologic Distress in Ambulatory Cancer Patients. *Cancer, 103 (7).* 1494–1502.
The method used in these reports to match distress scores with questionnaire scores plotted the receiver operating characteristic curves. I am passing on the details of that here.

[74] Lazenby, M., Dixon, J., Bai, M., & McCorkle, R. (2014) Comparing the Distress Thermometer With the Patient Health Questionnaire (PHQ)-2 for Screening for Possible Cases of Depression Among Patients Newly Diagnosed With Advanced Cancer. *Palliative & Supportive Care, 12 (01).* 63–68.

[75] Dawes, R.M.E. (1977) Suppose We Measured Height With Rating Scales Instead of Rulers. *Applied Psychological Measurement, 1 (2).* 267–273.

[76] Collet, C., Averty, P., & Dittmar, A. (2009) Autonomic Nervous System and Subjective Ratings of Strain in Air-traffic Control. *Applied Ergonomics, 40 (1).* 23–32.

[77] Nieder, A. (2020) Neural Constraints on Human Number Concepts. *Current Opinion in Neurobiology, 60.* 28–36.

[78] Shapiro, F. (1989) Eye Movement Desensitization: a New Treatment for Post-traumatic Stress Disorder. *Journal of Behavior Therapy & Experimental Psychiatry, 20 (3)*. 211–217.

[79] Shapiro, F. (1989) Efficacy of the Eye Movement Desensitization Procedure in the Treatment of Traumatic Memories. *Journal of Traumatic Stress, 2 (2)*. 199–223.

[80] Shapiro F. (2018) *Eye Movement Desensitization and Reprocessing Therapy* (3rd ed.). Guilford Publications.

[81] The stick is a length of hardwood 70cm long. Other dimensions can be those that comfortably fit the hand. The ends are rounded to prevent 'walking' when you use it. A target of some kind is glued to one end. On my stick there is a coin, which the patient is instructed to watch. It is pivoted on the therapist's seat, or somewhere else convenient to use. This avoids excessive effort in the therapist's right arm and shoulder. It also allows a change to the left side (or vice versa).

[82] The author uses the NeuroTek Tac/AudioScan (a signal box or 'buzz box'). Neurotec Corp, CO, USA. Other makes are available. There are android and iOS apps for this.

[83] (1.) Hornsveld, H.K., Hout veen, J.H., Vroomen, M., Aalbers, I.K.D., Aalbers, D., & van der Hout, M.A. (2011) Evaluating the Effect of Eye Movements on Positive Memories Such as Those Used in Resource Development and Installation. *Journal of EMDR Practice & Research, 5 (4)*. 146–155.

(2.) Leeds et al. (2011) Response to Hornsveld. *Journal of EMDR Practice & Research, 6 (4)*. 170–173,

(3.) Hornsveld et al. (2012) Reply to Leeds. *Journal of EMDR Practice & Research, 6 (4)*. 174–178.

[84] This value of one-third comes from an early and unpublished audit of my first 200 patients. I use this figure to warn my patients of the probability of distress recollection. However, the value comes from retrospectively reading notes and not all such events may have been recorded accurately. A distressing recollection can be named an abreaction. If we are to use this word then we should be aware that it carries historical meanings not necessarily suitable for eye movement desensitization.
Jackson S.W. (1994) Catharsis and Abreaction in the History of Psychological Healing. *Psychiatric Clinics of North America, 3*. 471–491.

[85] Hassard, A. (1993) Eye Movement Desensitization of Body Image. *Behavioural & Cognitive Psychotherapy, 21 (2)*. 157–160.

[86] Brown, K.W., McGoldrick, T., & Buchanan, R. (1997). Body Dysmorphic Disorder: Seven Cases Treated With Eye Movement Desensitization and Reprocessing. *Behavioural & Cognitive Psychotherapy, 25*. 203–208.

[87] Caputo, G.B. (2010) Strange-face-in-the mirror Illusion. *Perception, 39 (7)*. 1007–1008. doi.org/10.1068/p6466

[88] Henry, S.L. (1996) Pathological Gambling: Etiologic Considerations and Treatment Efficacy of Eye Movement Desensitization/Reprocessing. *Journal of Gambling Studies,* *12.* 395–405.

[89] Eimer, B.N., & Freeman, A. (1998) Reprocessing Pain Beliefs and Stressful Experiences. *Pain Management Psychotherapy. A Pract ical Guide.* John Wiley & Sons, New York, NY.

[90] Grant, M. (2001) Pain Control with Eye Movement Desensitization and Reprocessing. Mentor Books, Colorado, USA.

[91] Wilensky, M. (2006) Eye Movement Desensitization and Reprocessing (EMDR) as a Treatment for Phantom Limb Pain. *Journal of Brief Therapy, 5 (1).* 31–44.

[92] Schneider, J., Hofmann, A., Rost, C., & Shapiro, F. (2008) EMDR in the Treatment of Chronic Phantom Limb Pain. *Pain Medicine, 9 (1).* 76–82.

[93] Rostaminejad, M., Behnammoghadam, Z., Rost aminejada, M., Behnammoghadamc, Z., & Bashti, S. (2017) Efficacy of Eye Movement Desensitization and Reprocessing on the Phantom Limb Pain of Patients With Amputations Within a 24-month Follow-up.
International Journal of Rehabilitation Research, 40 (3). 209–214.

[94] Hase, M., Schallmayer, S., & Sack, M. (2008) EMDR Reprocessing of the Addiction Memory: Pre-treatment, Post-treatment, and 1-month Follow-up. *Journal of EMDR Practice & Research, 2 (3).* 170–179.

[95] Markus, W., & Hornsveld, H.K.(2017) EMDR Interventions in Addiction. *Journal of EMDR Practice & Research, 11 (1).* 3–29.

[96] Adler, S.R. (2011) *Sleep Paralysis.* Rutgers University Press.

[97] Denis, D., French, C.C., & Gregory, A.M. (2018) A Systematic Review of Variables Associated With Sleep Paralysis. *Sleep Medicine Reviews, 38.* 141–157.

[98] Van den Berg, D.P., Van der Vleugel, B.M., Staring, A.B., De Bont, P.A., & De Jongh, A. (2013). EMDR in Psychosis: Guidelines for Conceptualization and Treatment. *Journal of EMDR Practice & Research, 7.* 208–224.

[99] van den Berg, D.P., de Bont, P.A., van der Vleugel, B.M., de Roos, C., de Jongh, A., van Minnen, A., & van der Gaag, M. (2015) Prolonged Exposure vs Eye Movement Desensitization and Reprocessing vs Waiting List for Post-traumatic Stress Disorder in Patients With a Psychotic Disorder: a Randomized Clinical Trial. *JAMA Psychiatry, 72 (3).* 259–267.
The 12-month follow-up is: Long-term Outcomes of Trauma-focused Treatment in Psychosis. *The British Journal of Psychiatry (2018), 212 (3).* 180–182. This project suffers

from the issue to be discussed in Chapter 11. The prolonged exposure subjects get homework of listening to audio files of the event and therefore get more treatment time.

[100] Paris, J. (2012) The Rise and Fall of Dissociative Identity Disorder. *Journal of Nervous & Mental Disease, 200 (12).* 1076–1079.

[101] (1.) For the canonical account of diagnosis and treatment see:
(1.) International Society for the Study of Trauma & Dissociation (2011) Guidelines for Treating Dissociative Identity Disorder in Adults, (3rd revision). *Journal of Trauma Dissociation, 12.* 115–187.
(2.) For a colourful account of dissociative identity disorder treatment, including just how many alters can be found and how long treatment can last, see:
Kluft, R.P. (2013) *Shelter from the Storm.* www.createSpace.com
(3.) For this issue and eye movement therapy, see:
Gonzalez, A., Mosquera, D., et al. (2012) *EMDR & Dissociation: The Progressive Approach.* Amazon.co.uk

[102] For a critique, see the definitive reviews by:
(1.) Piper, A., & Merskey, H. (2004) The Persistence of Folly: a Critical Examination of Dissociative Identity Disorder. Part II. The Excesses of an Improbable Concept. *Canadian Journal of Psychiatry, 49.* 592–600.
(2) Piper, A., & Merskey, H. (2004) The Persistence of Folly: a

Critical Examination of Dissociative Identity Disorder. Part II. The Defence and Decline of Multiple Personality or Dissociative Identity Disorder. *Canadian Journal of Psychiatry, 49.* 678–1683.
(3) Piper, A. (1994). Multiple Personality Disorder. *The British Journal of Psychiatry, 164 (5).* 600–612.
(4) Lynn, S.J., Lilienfeld, S.O., Merckel-bach, H., Giesbrecht, T., & van der Kloet, D. (2012) Dissociation and Dissociative Disorders Challenging Conventional Wisdom. *Current Directions in Psychological Science, 21 (1).* 48–53.
(5) Shaffer, M.J., & Oakley, J.S. (2005) Some Epistemological Concerns About Dissociative Identity Disorder and Diagnostic Practices In Psychology. *Philosophical Psychology, 18.* 1–29.
(6) Molloy, C. (2015) "I just really love my spirit": A Rhetorical Inquiry Into Dissociative Identity Disorder. *Rhetoric Review, 34.* 462–478.

[103] Gunderson, J. (2009). Borderline Personality Disorder: Ontogeny of a Diagnosis. *American Journal of Psychiatry, 166 (5).* 530–539.

[104] Slotema, C.W., van den Berg, D.P., Driessen, A., Wilhelmus, B., & Franken, I.H. (2019) Feasibility of EMDR for Post-traumatic Stress Disorder in Patients With Personality Disorders: a Pilot Study. *European Journal of Psychotraumatology, 10 (1).* 1614822.

[105] Mosquera, D., Leeds, A.M., & Gonzalez, A. (2014). Application of EMDR Therapy for Borderline Personality Disorder. *Journal of EMDR Practice & Research, 8 (2).* 74.

[106] de Jongh, A., Ernst, R., Marques, L., & Hornsveld, H. (2013) The Impact of Eye Movements and Tones on Disturbing Memories Involving PTSD and Other Mental Disorders. *Journal of Behavior Therapy & Experimental Psychiatry, 44 (4).* 477–483.

[107] Ayala, E.S., Meuret, A.E., & Ritz, T. (2009) Treatments for Blood-injury-injection Phobia: a Critical Review of Current Evidence. *Journal of Psychiatric Research, 43 (15).* 1235–1242.

[108] For a discussion of this issue, see:
(1.) Greenwald, R. (2010) What is EMDR? Commentary by Greenwald. *Journal of EMDR Practice & Research, 4.* 170–179.
(2.) Shapiro, F. (2010) What is EMDR? Invited response by Shapiro. *Journal of EMDR Practice & Research, 5.* 25–28.

[109] Paul, G.L. (1967) Insight Versus Desensitization in Psychotherapy Two Years After Termination. *Journal of Consulting Psychology, 31.* 333–348.

[110] Cowan, N. (2005) *Working Memory Capacity.* Psychology Press.

[111] Richardson, J.T. (2007) Measures of Short-term Memory: a Historical Review. *Cortex, 43 (5).* 635–650.

[112] Jacobs, J. (1887) Experiments on "prehension". *Mind, 45.* 75–79. doi.org/10.1093/mind/os-12.45.75

[113] Miller, G.A. (1956) The Magical Number Seven, Plus or Minus Two: Some Limits on our Capacity for Processing Information. *Psychological Review, 63 (2).* 81–97. http://psychclassics.yorku.ca/Miller

[114] There may be a mathematical justification for the value of seven. Reports have been published showing that seven is an emergent property of the structure of neuron membranes or memory storage. I am too mathematically challenged to summarize this, but this helps to promotes seven as an important number for our purposes. For example, see Linhares, A., Chada, D.M., & Aranha C.N. (2011) The Emergence of Millers Magic Number on a Sparse Distribut ed Memory. *PLOS One, 6 (1).* e15592. doi.org/10.1371/journal.pone.0015592

[115] Changizi, M.A. (2008) Economically Organized Hierarchies in WordNet and the Oxford English Dictionary. *Cognitive Systems Research, 9 (3).* 214–228.

[116] Christophel, T.B., Klink, P.C., Spitzer, B., Roelfsema, P.R., & Haynes, J.D. (2017) The Distributed Nature of Working Memory. *Trends in Cognitive Sciences, 21 (2).*111 –124.

[117] Olivers, C.N., Peters, J., Houtkamp, R., & Roelfsema, P.R. (2011) Different States in Visual Working Memory: When it Guides Attention and When it Does Not. *Trends in Cognitive Sciences, 15.* 327–334.

[118] Cowan, N. (2010) The Magical Mystery Four: How is Working Memory Capacity Limited, and Why? *Current Directions in Psychological Science, 19.* 51–57.

[119] Hassard, A. (2003) Distribution of Targets in 400 Eye-Movement Desensitization Cases. *Psychological Reports, 92 (3).* 717–722.

[120] Hassard, A., Turner, H. & Smith, K. Dose Response and Working Memory Limit in an Eye Movement Desensitisation and Reprocessing Prospective Case Series. F1000Research. com (2018), 7:1471. doi.org/10.12688/f1000research.15648.1

[121] Moran, T.P. (2016) Anxiety and Working Memory Capacity: a Meta-analysis and Narrative Review. *Psychological Bulletin, 10.* 1–34. dx.doi.org/10.1037/bul0000051

[122] Hampshire, A., Highfield, R.R., Parkin, B.L., & Owen, A.M. (2012). Fractionating Human Intelligence. *Neuron, 76 (6).* 1225–1237.

[123] Scott, J.C., Matt, G.E., Wrocklage, K.M., Crnich, C., Jordan, J., Southwick, S.M., Krystald, J.H., & Schweinsburg, B.C. (2015). A Quantitative Meta-analysis of Neurocognitive Functioning in Post-traumatic Stress Disorder. Psychological Bulletin, 141 (1). 105–140. doi.org/10.1037/a0038039

[124] Leach, J., & Griffith, R. (2008) Restrictions in Working Memory Capacity During Parachuting: a Possible Cause of

"No Pull" Fatalities. *Applied Cognitive Psychology, 22 (2).* 147–157.

[125] Moriya, J., & Sugiura, Y. (2012) High Visual Working Memory Capacity in Trait Social Anxiety. *PLOS One, 7 (4).* e34244.

[126] Postle, B.R., Idzikowski, C., Sala, S.D., Logie, R.H., & Baddeley, A.D. (2006) The Selective Disruption of Spatial Working Memory by Eye Movements. *The Quarterly Journal of Experimental Psychology, 59 (1).* 100–120.

[127] Theeuwes, J., Belopolsky, A., & Olivers, C.N. (2009) Interactions Between Working Memory, Attention and Eye Movements. *Acta Psychologica, 132 (2).* 106–114.

[128] Crick, F., & Mitchison, G. (1986) REM Sleep and Neural Nets. *Journal of Mind & Behavior, 7.* 229–249.

[129] (1.) Tryon, W.W. (1999) A Bidirectional Associative Memory Explanation of Post-traumatic Stress Disorder. *Clinical Psychology Review, 19 (7).* 789–818.
(2.) Tryon, W.W. (2005). Possible Mechanisms for Why Desensitization and Exposure Therapy Work. *Clinical Psychology Review, 25 (1).* 67–95.
(3.) Tryon, W.W. (2012). A Connectionist Network Approach to Psychological Science: Core and Corollary Principles. *Review of General Psychology, 16 (3).* 305.

[130] Tyler, W.J. (2012) The Mechanobiology of Brain Function. *Nature Reviews Neuroscience, 13 (12)*. 867–878.

[131] Hameroff, S., & Penrose, R. (2013) Consciousness in the Universe: a Review of the "Orch OR" Theory. *Physics of Life Reviews, 11 (1)*. 39–78.

[132] Hassard, A. (1996). Reverse Learning and the Physiological Basis of Eye Movement Desensitization. *Medical Hypotheses, 47 (4)*. 277–282.

[133] Silber, M.H., & 12 others (2007). The Visual Scoring of Sleep in Adults. *Journal of Clinical Sleep Medicine, 3 (2)*. 121–131.

[134] Goldstein, A.N., & Walker, M.P. (2014) The Role of Sleep in Emotional Brain Function. *Annual Review of Clinical Psychology, 10*. 679–708.

[135] Diekelmann, S., & Born, J. (2010) The Memory Function of Sleep. *Nature Reviews Neuroscience, 11 (2)*. 114–126.

[136] Conte, F., & Ficca, G. (2013) Caveats on Psychological Models of Sleep and Memory: a Compass in an Overgrown Scenario. *Sleep Medicine Reviews, 17 (2)*. 105–121.

[137] Axmacher, N., Draguhn, A., Elger, C.E., & Fell, J. (2009) Memory Processes During Sleep: Beyond the Standard Consolidation Theory. *Cellular & Molecular Life Sciences, 66 (14)*. 2285–2297.

[138] Pace-Schott, E.F., Germain, A., & Milad, M.R. (2015) Sleep and REM Sleep Disturbance in the Pathophysiology of PTSD: the Role of Extinction Memory. *Biology of Mood & Anxiety Disorders, 5 (1).* 3.

[139] Landmann, N., Kuhn, M., Maier, J.G., Spiegelhalder, K., Baglioni, C., Frasea, L., Riemanna D., Sterrb A., & Nissen, C. (2015). REM Sleep and Memory Reorganisation: Potential Relevance for Psychiatry and Psychotherapy. *Neurobiology of Learning & Memory, 122.* 28–40. doi.org/10.1016/j.nlm.2015.01.004

[140] Callaway, C.W., Lydic, R., Baghdoyan, H.A., & Hobson, J.A. (1987) Pontogeniculooccipital Waves: Spontaneous Visual System Activity During Rapid Eye Movement Sleep. *Cellular & Molecular Neurobiology, 7 (2).* 105–149.

[141] Datta, S. (1997) Cellular Basis of Pontine Ponto-geniculo-occipital Wave Generation and Modulation. *Cellular & Molecular Neurobiology, 17 (3).* 341–365.

[142] Stuart, K., & Conduit, R. (2009) Auditory Inhibition of Rapid Eye Movements and Dream Recall from REM Sleep. *Sleep, 32 (3).* 399–408.

[143] Lim, A.S., Lozano, A.M., Moro, E., Hamani, C., Hutchison, W.D., Dostrovsky, J.O., Lang, A.E., Wennberg, R.A. & Murray, B.J. (2007) Characterization of REM Sleep Associated Ponto-geniculo-occipital Waves in the Human Pons. *Sleep, 30 (7).* 823–827.

[144] Fernández-Mendoza, J., Lozano, B., Seijo, F., Santamarta-Liébana, E., Ramos-Plat ón, M. J., Vela-Bueno, A., & Fernández-González, F. (2009) Evidence of Subthalamic PGO-like Waves During REM Sleep in Humans: a Deep Brain Polysomnographic Study. *Sleep, 32 (9).* 1117–1126.

[145] Andrillon, T., Nir, Y., Cirelli, C., Tononi, G., & Fried, I. (2015) Single-neuron Activity and Eye Movements During Human REM Sleep and Awake Vision. *Nature Communications, 6.* 1–10.

[146] Bowker, R.M. & Morrison, A.R. (1966) The Startle Reflex and PGO Spikes. *Brain Research, 102 (1).* 185–190.

[147] Donaldson, I.M.L. (2000) The Functions of the Proprioceptors of the Eye Muscles. Philosophical Transactions of the Royal Society of London. *Series B: Biological Sciences, 355 (1404).* 1685.

[148] Datta, S., & O'Malley, M.W. (2013) Fear Extinction Memory Consolidation Requires Potentiation of Pontine-wave Activity During REM Sleep. *The Journal of Neuroscience, 33 (10).* 4561–4569.

[149] Gross, J., Byrne, J. & Fisher, C. (1965) Eye Movements During Emergent Stage 1 EEG in Subjects With Lifelong Blindness. *Journal of Nervous & Mental Disease, 141 (3).* 365–370.

[150] Wilson, S., & Argyropoulos, S. (2005). Antidepressants and Sleep. *Drugs, 65 (7).* 927–947.

[151] Nir, Y., & Tononi, G. (2010) Dreaming and the Brain: from Phenomenology to Neurophysiology. *Trends in Cognitive Sciences, 14 (2).* 88–100.

[152] Wamsley, E.J., & Stickgold, R. (2011) Memory, Sleep, and Dreaming: Experiencing Consolidation. *Sleep Medicine Clinics, 6 (1).* 97–108.

[153] Pizza, F., Fabbri, M., Magosso, E., Ursino, M., Provini, F., Ferri, R., & Montagna, P. (2011) Slow Eye Movements Distribution During Nocturnal Sleep. *Clinical Neurophysiology, 122 (8).* 1556–1561.

[154] Lencer, R., & Trillenberg, P. (2008) Neurophysiology and Neuroanatomy of Smooth Pursuit in Humans. *Brain & Cognition, 68 (3).* 219–228.

[155] McDowell, J.E., Dyckman, K.A., Austin, B.P., & Clementz, B.A. (2008) Neurophysiology and Neuroanatomy of Reflexive and Volitional Saccades: Evidence from Studies of Humans. *Brain & Cognit ion, 68 (3).* 255–270. doi.org/10.1016/j.bandc.2008.08.016

[156] Sun, L.D., & Goldberg, M.E. (2016) Corollary Discharge and Oculomotor Proprioception: Cortical Mechanisms for Spatially Accurate Vision. *Annual Review of Vision Science, 2.* 61–84.

[157] Wang, J., & Pan, Y. (2013) Eye Proprioception May Provide Real Time Eye Position Information. *Neurological Sciences, 34 (3).* 281–286.

[158] Lebranchu, P., Bastin, J., Pélégrini-Issac, M., Lehericy, S., Berthoz, A., & Orban, GA. (2010) Retinotopic Coding of Extraretinal Pursuit Signals in Early Visual Cortex. *Cerebral Cortex, 20 (9).* 2172–2187.

[159] Buzsaki, G. (2006) *Rhythms of the Brain.* New York: Oxford University Press.

[160] Niedermeyer, E., & da Silva, F.L. (eds.) (2005) *Electroencephalography: Basic Principles, Clinical Applications, and Related Fields.* Lippincott Williams & Wilkins.
Mostly from Chapter 9, *The Normal EEG of the Waking Adult* by E. Niedermeyer; and Chapter 10, *Sleep and EEG* by E. Niedermeyer. To give you an indication of the size of this subject, this book measures 28 × 22 × 6.5cm and weighs 3kg.

[161] Bazanova, O.M., & Vernon, D. (2014) Interpreting EEG Alpha Activity. *Neuroscience & Biobehavioral Reviews, 44.* 94–110.

[162] Romei, V., Gross, J., & Thut, G. (2012) Sounds Reset Rhythms of Visual Cortex and Corresponding Human Visual Perception. *Current Biology, 22 (9).* 807–813.

[163] Colgin, L.L. (2013) Mechanisms and Functions of Theta Rhythms. *Annual Review of Neuroscience, 36.* 295–312.

[164] Cowdin, N., Kobayashi, I., & Mellman, T.A. (2014) Theta Frequency Activity During Rapid Eye Movement Sleep is Greater in People With Resilience Versus PTSD. *Experimental Brain Research, 232 (5).* 1479–1485.

[165] Bastin, J., Lebranchu, P., Jerbi, K., Kahane, P., Orban, G., Lachaux, J.P., & Berthoz, A. (2012) Direct Recordings in Human Cortex Reveal the Dynamics of Gamma-band [50–150 hz] Activity During Pursuit Eye Movement Control. *Neuroimage, 63 (1).* 339–347.

[166] Huber, R., Ghilardi, M.F., Massimini, M., Ferrarelli, F., Riedner, B.A., Peterson, M.J., & Tononi, G. (2006) Arm Immobilization Causes Cortical Plastic Changes and Locally Decreases Sleep Slow Wave Activity. *Nature Neuroscience, 9 (9).* 1169–1176.

[167] Clawson, B.C., Durkin, J., & At on, S.J. (2016) Form and Function of Sleep Spindles Across the Lifespan. Neural Plasticity. dx.doi.org/10.1155/2016/6936381

[168] Lindemann, C., Ahlbeck, J., Bitzenhofer, S.H., & Hanganu-Opatz, I.L. (2016) Spindle Activity Orchestrates Plasticity During Development and Sleep. *Neural Plasticity.* dx.doi.org/10.1155/2016/5787423

[169] Achermann, P., Rusterholz, T., Dürr, R., König, T., & Tarokh, L. (2016) Global Field Synchronization Reveals Rapid Eye Movement Sleep as Most Synchronized Brain State in the Human EEG. *Royal Society Open Science*, 3 (10).160201.

[170] Simor, P., van Der Wijk, G., Gombos, F., & Kovács, I. (2019) The Paradox of Rapid Eye Movement Sleep in the Light of Oscillatory Activity and Cortical Synchronization During Phasic and Tonic Microstates. *NeuroImage, 202.* 116066.

[171] Simor, P., van der Wijk, G., Nobili, L., & Peigneux, P. (2020) The Microstructure of REM Sleep: Why Phasic and Tonic. *Sleep Medicine Reviews.* 101305.

[172] Pagani, M., Högberg, G., Fernandez, I., & Siracusano, A. (2013) Correlates of EMDR Therapy in Functional and Structural Neuroimaging: a Critical Summary of Recent Findings. *Journal of EMDR Practice & Research, 7 (1).* 29–38.

[173] Pagani, M., Di Lorenzo, G., Verardo, A.R., Nicolais, G., Monaco, L., Lauretti, G., Russo, R., Niolu, N., Ammaniti, M., Fernandez, I., & Siracusano, A. (2012) Neurobiological Correlates of EMDR Monitoring an EEG St udy. *PLOS one, 7 (9).* e45753.

[174] Elofsson, U.O., von Schéele, B., Theorell, T., & Söndergaard, H.P. (2008) Physiological Correlates of Eye Movement Desensitization and Reprocessing. *Journal of Anxiety Disorders, 22 (4).* 622–634.

[175] Pagani, M., Högberg, G., Salmaso, D., Nardo, D., Sundin, Ö., Jonsson, C., Soares, J., Åberg-Wistedt, A., Jacobsson, H., Larsson, S.A., & Hällström, T. (2007) Effects of EMDR Psychotherapy on 99mTc-HMPAO Distribution in Occupation-related Post-traumatic Stress Disorder. *Nuclear Medicine Communications, 28 (10)*. 757–765.

[176] Bossini, L., Santarnecchi, E., Casolaro, I., Koukouna, D., Caterini, C., Cecchini, Fortini, V., Vatti, G., Marino, D., Fernandez, I., & Rossi, A. (2017). Morphovolumetric Changes After EMDR Treatment in Drug-naïve PTSD Patients. *Rivista Di Psichiatria, 52 (1)*. 24–31.

[177] Laugharne, J., Kullack, C., Lee, C. W., McGuire, T., Brockman, S., Drummond, P.D., & Starkstein, S. (2016) Amygdala Volumetric Change Following Psychotherapy for Post-traumatic Stress Disorder. *The Journal of Neuropsychiatry & Clinical Neuro Sciences, 28*. 312–318. doi.org/10.1176/appi.neuropsych.16010006

[178] Craig, A.D. (2015) *How Do You Feel? An Interoceptive Moment With Your Neurobiological Self.* Princeton University Press.
This is a somewhat dense but informative account of the relevant physiology.

[179] Colombi, I., Tinarelli, F., Pasquale, V., Tucci, V., & Chiappalone, M. (2016) A Simplified in Vitro Experimental Model Encompasses the Essential Features of Sleep. *Frontiers in Neuroscience, 10*. 315. doi.org/10.3389/fnins.2016.00315

[180] Lindquist, K.A., Wager, T.D., Kober, H., Bliss-Moreau, E., & Barrett, L.F. (2012) The Brain Basis of Emotion: a Meta-analytic Review. *Behavioral & Brain Sciences, 35 (3)*. 121–143.

[181] Hart, D., & Sussman, R.W. (2005) *Man the Hunted: Primates, Predators, and Humans.* Westview Press, Perseus Books.

[182] Lieberman, D.E., Bramble, D.M., Raichlen, D.A., & Shea, J.J. (2009) Brains, Brawn, and the Evolution of Human Endurance Running Capabilities. *The First Humans? Origin and Early Evolut ion of the Genus Homo.* 77–92. Springer, Netherlands.

[183] Robert, V.A., & Casadevall, A. (2009) Vertebrate Endothermy Restricts Most Fungi as Potential Pathogens. *Journal of Infectious Diseases, 200 (10).* 1623–1626.

[184] Rial, R.V., Nicolau, M.C.,Gamundí, A., Akaârir, M., Aparicio, S., Garau, C., Tejada, S., Roca, C., Gené, L., Moranta, D., & Esteban,S. (2007) The Trivial Function of Sleep. *Sleep Medicine Reviews, 11 (4).* 311–325.

[185] Rial, R.V., Akaârir, M., Gamundí, A., Nicolau, C., Garau, C., Aparicio, S., Tejada, S., Gené, L., González, J., De Vera, L.M. (2010) Evolution of Wakefulness, Sleep and Hibernation: from Reptiles to Mammals. *Neuroscience & Biobehavioral Reviews, 34 (8).* 1144–1160.

[186] Schmitz, L., & Motani, R. (2011) Nocturnality in Dinosaurs Inferred from Scleral Ring and Orbit Morphology. *Science, 332 (6030).* 705–708.

[187] Angielczyk, K.D., & Schmitz L. (2014) Nocturnality in Synapsids Predates the Origin of Mammals by over 100 Million Years. *Proceedings of the Royal Society B: Biological Sciences, 281 (1793).* 20141642.

[188] Blumberg, M.S., Lesku, J.A., Libourel, P.A., Schmidt, M.H., & Rattenborg, N.C. (2020). What Is REM Sleep? *Current Biology, 30 (1).* R38-R49.

[189] Horne, J. (2013). Why REM sleep? Clues Beyond the Laboratory in a More Challenging World. *Biological Psychology, 92 (2).* 152–168.

[190] Valli, K., & Revonsuo, A. (2009) The Threat Simulation Theory in Light of Recent Empirical Evidence: a Review. *American Journal of Psychology.* 17–38.

[191] Preston, B.T., Capellini, I., McNamara, P., Barton, R.A., & Nunn, C.L. (2009) Parasite Resistance and the Adaptive Significance of Sleep. *BMC Evolut ionary Biology, 9 (1).* doi.org/10.1186/1471-2148-9-7

[192] Ekirch, A.R. (2000) Sleep we Have Lost: Pre-indust rial Slumber in the British Isles. *The American Historical Review, 106 (2).* 343–386.

[193] Wehr, T.A. (1992) In Short Photoperiods, Human Sleep is Biphasic. *Journal of Sleep Research, 1 (2)*. 103–107.

[194] Isbell, L.A. (2006) Snakes as Agents of Evolutionary Change in Primate Brains. *Journal of Human Evolution, 51 (1)*. 1–35.

[195] Isbell, L.A. (2009). *The Fruit, the Tree, and the Serpent.* Harvard University Press.

[196] de Jongh, A., Amann, B.L., Hofmann, A., Farrell, D., & Lee, C.W. (2019) The Status of EMDR Therapy in the Treatment of Post-traumatic Stress Disorder 30 Years After its Introduction. *Journal of EMDR Practice & Research, 13 (4)*. 261–269.

[197] Stanbury, M., Drummond, P.D., Laugharne, J., Kullack, C., & Lee, C.W. (2020) Comparative Efficiency of EMDR and Prolonged Exposure in Treating Post-traumatic Stress Disorder: a Randomized Trial. *Journal of EMDR Practice & Research, 14 (1)*. 2–12.

[198] Leung, L. (2012) Pain Catastrophizing: an Updated Review. *Indian Journal of Psychological Medicine, 34 (3)*. 204–217.

[199] Philips, H.C. (2011) Imagery and Pain: the Prevalence, Characteristics, and Potency of Imagery Associated With Pain. *Behavioural & Cognitive Psychotherapy, 39 (5)*. 523–540.

[200] Philips, H.C., & Samson, D. (2012). The Rescripting of Pain Images. *Behavioural & Cognitive Psychotherapy, 40 (5)*. 558–576. doi.org/10.1017/S1352465812000549

[201] Tesarz, J., Wicking, M., Bernardy, K., & Seidler, G.H. (2019) EMDR Therapy's Efficacy in the Treatment of Pain. *Journal of EMDR Practice & Research, 13 (4)*. 337–344. connect.springerpub.com/content/sgremdr/13/4/337

[202] Marcus, S.V. (2008) Phase 1 of Integrated EMDR: An Abortive Treatment for Migraine Headaches. *Journal of EMDR Practice & Research, 2 (1)*. 15–25.

[203] Gerhardt, A., Leisner, S., Hartmann, M., Janke, S., Seidler, G.H., Eich, W., & Tesarz, J. (2016) Eye Movement Desensitization and Reprocessing vs. Treatment-as-usual for Non-specific Chronic Back Pain Patients With Psychological Trauma: a Randomized Controlled Pilot Study. *Frontiers in Psychiatry, 7*. 201. doi.org/10.3389/fpsyt.2016.00201

[204] Majorek, M. (2012) Does the Brain Cause Conscious Experience? *Journal of Consciousness Studies, 19 (3–4)*. 121–144.

[205] Forsdyke, D.R. (2015) Wittgensteins Certainty is Uncertain: Brain Scans of Cured Hydrocephalics Challenge Cherished Assumptions. *Biological Theory, 10 (4)*. 336–342.

[206] McFie, J. (1961) The Effects of Hemispherectomy on

Intellectual Functioning in Cases of Infantile Hemiplegia. *Journal of Neurology, Neurosurgery & Psychiatry, 24 (3).* 240–248.

[207] Devlin, A.M., Cross, J.H., Harkness, W., Chong, W.K., Harding, B., Vargha-Khadem, F., & Neville, B.G.R. (2003) Clinical Outcomes of Hemispherectomy for Epilepsy in Childhood and Adolescence. *Brain, 126 (3).* 556–566.

[208] Harris, J., (2017) Rewiring Neuroscience. www.rewiring-neuroscience.com. Last checked March 2021.

[209] Furedi, F. (2004) *Therapy Culture: Cultivating Vulnerability in an Uncertain Age.* Routledge Press.

[210] There are many reports on the varying effects of child abuse, not pursued here. You might like to start with: Clancy, S.A. (2009) *The Trauma Myth.* Basic Books.

[211] Frueh, B.C., Elhai, J.D., Grubaugh, A.L., Monnier, J., Kashdan, T.B., Sauvageot, J.A., & Arana, G.W. (2005) Documented Combat Exposure of US Veterans Seeking Treatment for Combat-related Post-traumatic Stress Disorder. *British Journal of Psychiatry, 186 (6).* 467–472.

[212] Savino, J.O., & Turvey, B.E. (eds.) (2011) False Allegations of Sexual Assault. *Rape Investigation Handbook.* Academic Press.

[213] Eastwood, S., & Bisson, J.I. (2008) Management of Factitious Disorders: a Systematic Review. *Psychotherapy & Psychosomatics, 77 (4).* 209–218.

[214] Fardin M.A. (2020) COVID-19 and Anxiety: A Review of Psychological Impacts of Infectious Disease Outbreaks. Archives of Clinical Infectious Diseases. 15(COVID-19):e102779. doi:10.5812/archcid.102779

INDEX

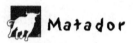

For exclusive discounts on Matador titles,
sign up to our occasional newsletter at
troubador.co.uk/bookshop